YOUR SMILE, YOUR HEALTH, YOUR SUCCESS

CONTRIBUTIONS BY AMERICA'S PREMIER ORTHODONTISTS

Your Smile, Your Health, Your Success
Contributions by America's Premier Orthodontists

ISBN 978-0-9905746-5-1

CONTENTS

INTRODUCTION
THE IMPORTANCE OF A STUNNING SMILE
DR. BARRY GLASER

"We shall never know all the good that a simple smile can do."
Mother Teresa

For better or worse, the way we present ourselves to the world matters. Whether in social situations or the boardroom, it's important to put our best foot forward. An area that should not be overlooked is a winning smile.

It has been said that you only get one chance at making a good first impression, and in those first critical moments everything counts! A firm handshake, confident eye contact, and a dazzling smile all provide nonverbal cues that we have the "right stuff". In an increasingly competitive world, we must make the most of every advantage – and a stunning smile is just what the doctor ordered!

Numerous studies and statistics show that smiling plays an integral role in making that successful first impression. According to the *Forbes* article "Seven Seconds to Make a

First Impression," your smile is part of nonverbal positive signals that either invite people in or possibly repel them away. The article said, "A smile is an invitation, a sign of welcome. It says, 'I'm friendly and approachable.'"

Not only is smiling important, but also what you reveal with your smile plays another critical role in overall positive perception and response – your teeth.

According to the *PR News Wire* article, "First Impressions Are Everything: New Study Confirms People With Straight Teeth Are Perceived as More Successful, Smarter and Having More Dates," teeth are critical to perception. *The Kelton Survey,* which was conducted by Invisalign®, said, "Findings back up the negative judgments about people with crooked teeth; two in five Americans would not go on a second date with someone who has crooked teeth and more than half believe someone with crooked teeth would be less likely to land a job when competing with someone who has a similar skill set and experience."

Most people don't want to admit that something like crooked or stained teeth could convince them not to date a person or even hire him or her, but these studies confirm what many of us don't want to confess: an embarrassing smile of any kind can hold people back in life.

Let's take for example Dr. Barry Glaser's patient, "Peter" (not his real name) a 40-year-old male who presented for treatment. Peter had very little dental care up to that point, and since Dr. Glaser referred him to a local dentist for extensive dental work prior to orthodontic treatment, he had the opportunity to get to know him.

Peter was unemployed, still lived with his parents, appeared unkempt, and was mildly depressed. As he progressed through gum treatment, extractions and fillings, he would occasionally meet at Dr. Glaser's office so that the doctor could re-evaluate his dental condition. After some time, his dental condition was stabilized, and he began orthodontic treatment in Dr. Glaser's office. His treatment lasted approximately two years.

As is routine in every case at Dr. Glaser's office, before and after photographs were obtained. It wasn't until Dr. Glaser evaluated his before and after photos that he was truly struck by the physical transformation Peter went through. In addition to his handsome new smile, he had lost close to 100 pounds, his hair was neatly cut; he was clean shaven and was dressed in a suit and tie.

At his first retainer-check visit, Dr. Glaser commented to the patient about his metamorphosis. Peter related to Dr. Glaser and his staff that he was gainfully employed, had moved into his own apartment, and was in a relationship for the first time in decades. Dr. Glaser was astounded when Peter told him that all of this wouldn't have been possible if he hadn't become his patient. He told the doctor that in retrospect, he was so terribly self-conscious about his unsightly smile that it affected all other aspects of his life. Taking the first step to improving his smile led to a huge boost in self-confidence and completely changed the course of his life!

As is evidenced by the transformation of Peter, a great smile boosts self-confidence. His story is very common after patients have sought orthodontic treatment and enjoyed beautiful results.

"An individual's self-concept is the core of his personality. It affects every aspect of human behavior: the ability to learn, the capacity to grow and change. A strong, positive self-image is the best possible preparation for success in life."

Dr Joyce Brothers

The inward feeling of confidence a person feels when he or she knows they have a winning smile not only boosts his or her feelings of self-worth, it also reflects outwardly. Humans gravitate toward winners – whether it's the innate need to associate with those who are successful or a conscious desire to be with confident, successful individuals, everyone loves a winner!

Imagine waking up on a gloomy Monday morning. Maybe you hate your job, or you're in a failing relationship. You just want to turn off the alarm and go back to sleep. Now imagine feeling like that every day! When one isn't confident in his or her appearance this is how he or she may feel. When this person looks in the mirror and opens his or her mouth and all he or she sees are crooked or protruding teeth, inwardly this can do damage. Buck teeth, crooked teeth or other bite problems – all of these issues can hurt self-confidence. In fact, a person might feel so bad about his or her smile and teeth, he or she won't even confidently smile, and when the person does he or she might use a hand to cover up that smile. Ever see someone do this? It's not inviting, is it?

Now contrast those feelings with the way you might feel when you wake up on the first day of a great vacation. You can't wait to get out of bed and take on all the exciting possibilities of a new day. If you could bottle that feeling – summon it on demand – perhaps at the moment you first meet a blind date or enter the boardroom – is there anything that isn't possible? Confidence in one's appearance is the foundation of overall self-confidence.

Self-confidence and greater self-esteem project to the world we are successful and attract even more success in everything we do. Think about it. Have you ever seen a CEO give a presentation or speech where you thought he or she weren't self-confident or had high self-esteem. When you lack self-confidence and don't value yourself others won't value you either. You project this to the world, and others see it. In professional relationships if you don't stand up for yourself or speak with authority, you can be overlooked, underpaid, or passed up for promotions. Even in personal relationships when you don't value yourself or think you're worth something you are far more likely to fall into an abusive situation or be treated poorly.

It only makes sense that starting with something as fixable as your teeth could be your first step in changing your life just like the 40-year-old patient.

WHAT ARE WE FIXING?

Problems with teeth go beyond just crooked teeth. Many different issues related to your teeth and bite exist. The good news is that all of it can be fixed by seeing an orthodontist. You don't have to accept or live with your teeth problems.

Here are the various issues with teeth:

Crooked Teeth. Crooked teeth can harbor more bacterial plaque, which may lead to an increased risk for tooth decay and periodontal (gum) disease. Bacterial plaque is composed of living micro-organisms that eat sugars and other carbohydrates and produce many toxic waste products that are directly linked to dental disease. In addition, there is a growing body of evidence that links gum disease to other chronic diseases in the human body such as heart disease. By straightening the teeth, the risks of devastating dental diseases is reduced.

Overbites. In addition to being unsightly, overbites may lead to traumatic occlusion – the term orthodontists use to describe teeth that are hitting abnormally hard. Traumatic occlusion can lead to such problems as abnormal tooth wear, chipping or cracking of the teeth, loosening of the teeth, and potentially ultimately untimely tooth loss. In addition, research has shown that children with large overbites may be more prone to dental injury – fracturing or knocking out teeth – during sports or at play.

Crossbites. Crossbites may be anterior – in the front teeth, posterior – in the back teeth, or both. Crossbites may lead to abnormal tooth wear, direct-biting trauma to the teeth in crossbite, or serious gum problems where the tooth in crossbite is literally forced out of the gums. The American Association of Orthodontists recommends all children receive an orthodontic screening exam by age seven. Why? By age seven, the permanent teeth are beginning to erupt, and the orthodontist can assess if there are any bite issues that require early intervention. Crossbite correction is one of the issues that benefit from early intervention. While a seven- or eight-year old responds quite well to simple crossbite correction, adults with similar crossbites may require corrective jaw surgery!

Underbites. Underbites, where the lower teeth jut out further than the upper teeth can lead to serious issues. Abnormal tooth wear, poor chewing, and an unsightly smile are just some of the problems. In many cases, an underbite may be caused by abnormal growth of the jaws – another reason to have your child evaluated by an orthodontist by age seven. Jaw surgery is often indicated in severe cases of underbite.

Close Gaps in Teeth. One of the most common reasons for patients to seek orthodontic treatment are spaces between the teeth. While generally not a serious health issue, large gaps between the teeth can ruin an otherwise beautiful smile.

Teeth-lips alignment. You may not realize that your lips are supported by your teeth. If the teeth stick out too far, the lips may appear abnormally full. On the other hand, if the teeth lean in too far, the lips may be under-supported. This leads to thinning and wrinkling of the lips and will prematurely age you. Not good at all!

A HEALTHY SMILE'S VALUE TO THE PERSON'S LIFE

When you put the whole picture together, the question whether or not you should seek orthodontic treatment is clear – absolutely. A beautiful smile is truly more than skin deep. Having a beautiful smile boosts one's self-esteem and self-confidence. In addition, there are numerous health benefits both in the mouth as well as in the rest of the body.

Orthodontic treatment is truly one of the best investments one can make in themselves. There are treatment options available today such as clear braces and invisible removable aligners that make orthodontic treatment easier and more comfortable than ever. New technologies such as 3-D digital scanning, digital radiography, and computer-assisted treatment help make treatment predictable and efficient. Most orthodontists offer flexible payment options to help make treatment fit into most budgets, and many insurance companies help cover a percentage of the cost.

As you read through this book and hear about each of the new treatment options and technologies, you will be able to better decide what would work best for you. The question isn't would you want orthodontic treatment, it's why *wouldn't* you want orthodontic treatment?

CHAPTER 1
WHAT IS AN ORTHODONTIST?
DR. BARRY GLASER

"Wrinkles should merely indicate where smiles have been."
Mark Twain

Smiling, happy faces! Who doesn't appreciate being welcomed or greeted with a broad, beautiful smile? What happens though when that same greeting is somehow marred by a tight, uncomfortable smile or even a solemn nod? Is the feeling or response toward the person the same? Generally speaking most people react very positively to a smile versus a serious look or nod, which can elicit caution or concern instead of warmth and optimism.

What if the reason the person isn't smiling has nothing to do with his or her mood or feelings of happiness or kindness toward the other person? What if that bright, shining smile isn't on the person's face because he or she feels self-conscious about his or her teeth? They don't want to show the world what is embarrassing or makes them feel they need to hide something in their mouths – imperfect teeth.

Does this sound like an extreme reaction to crooked teeth? Maybe to someone who feels all right or even great about his or her teeth this behavior might seem too much or even ridiculous. Truth is, if you've ever felt uncomfortable with your teeth – whether crooked, bucked or somehow misaligned – it might be difficult to relate to those self-conscious feelings, but for the person who suffers with it, those feelings are real.

Many adults, children or teens, who don't feel pride about their teeth, often don't react positively to something that comes easily and naturally to most people (smiling). They sometimes don't want to expose what's bothering them. In fact, some people are so troubled about their teeth that when they do smile, they may even keep their lips closed or use their hands to cover up that smile.

Just as important as an attractive smile is having teeth that are aligned in a healthy bite. A "malocclusion" (literally meaning "bad bite") can adversely affect the health, stability, function and longevity of the teeth. The teeth should ideally fit together in a Class I occlusion – where the upper and lower teeth mesh together. Picture how the teeth of gears fit together – interlocking perfectly. Now imagine the consequences if the gears do not line up properly. The teeth of the gears will become prematurely worn down or may fracture completely from the abnormal stresses placed on them. In cases of severe misalignment, the gears may become seized and will not function at all.

It's the same with teeth. Misalignment of the teeth may lead to abnormal wear, fracture, *abfractions* – cracking or notching at the necks of the teeth or premature loosening of the teeth. The orthodontist takes the long-term health of the teeth and supporting structures into consideration when determining a treatment plan for a patient just as much as the esthetics of the smile.

Today no one need cover his or her smile! Orthodontists can help many of their patients achieve a healthy bite and beautiful smile!

WHAT IS AN ORTHODONTIST?

Who fixes those teeth? Orthodontists. An orthodontist is a specialist in the diagnosis, prevention and treatment of improper positioning of the teeth and facial structures. All orthodontists are dentists, however only six percent of dentists are orthodontists.

A general definition of an orthodontist is a person who is a type of dentist who specializes in treating and straightening crooked teeth. A dentist specializes in health care of the mouth, including treatment of mouth disease, filling of cavities, or repairing of teeth. On the other hand, an orthodontist's focus is to design brace-type systems (now including the latest technology like Invisalign® that features invisible aligners) to straighten teeth.

How did the profession of orthodontist come about? The occupation dates back much further than most people may realize. Archeologists have discovered Greek and Etruscan orthodontic relics dating to as early as 1000 BC. Around 400 BC, Hippocrates was one of the first to describe irregularities of the teeth. In 1728, French physician Pierre Fauchard published the first dental textbook in which he described an appliance designed to correct irregularities of the teeth. In 1878 Norman Kingsley published one of the first textbooks that deals specifically with straightening the teeth.

However, it was Edward Hartley Angle who is considered to be the "father of American orthodontics". In 1900, he formally established orthodontics as the first official specialty of dentistry. Angle coined the term "malocclusion," literally meaning "bad bite," and developed a system of classification of malocclusion that is still used today.

He also invented appliances to straighten the teeth that are the precursor to modern orthodontic braces. The original orthodontic treatments you may remember from the 60's and 70's were the big, clunky and ugly metal bands glued with dental cement. Since individual bands went around each individual tooth like a ring on a finger, it often resulted in more mouth and tongue sores, pain and discomfort. Wire was threaded through each bracket, and the teeth moved steadily by force.

External appliances such as headgears were more necessary and commonplace. Many children often endured jeers of peers who found braces and headgears something to target and make fun of. Embarrassed children were less likely to wear their headgears, which only impeded results and prolonged the process. When the braces were removed sometimes the cement adhesive didn't come easily off and tooth enamel might be adversely affected.

In the 70's, major advances in the field of orthodontics included the development of adhesives, which allowed for the first time, the direct bonding of a metal brace to the front surface of the tooth and greatly reduced the need for metal bands wrapped around each tooth. Another stride came around the same time. In the 80's, the development of super elastic nickel titanium "shape-memory" wires contributed to making orthodontic treatment more efficient, accurate and comfortable.

Improved adhesives, brackets and shape-memory wires combined gave rise to the "straight-wire" system of orthodontics. Advancements in shape memory and the advantages of new adhesives helped create this revolutionary method. More recently, "self-ligating" braces – where a wire is directly clipped into the brace – have been developed that allowed wires to seamlessly slide through. Think about it like threading beads. You slide a wire through each brace to create a chain-like effect. Next time you see someone with braces in their mouths, look carefully. Chances are this person probably has this type of braces on their teeth.

Now with this new methodology and improved adhesives problems of the past, among them mouth sores generated from friction on the inside of the bands near the tongue became less prevalent. Self-ligating systems provide overall easier movement of the teeth, improved oral hygiene with the ability to brush and floss easier, and reported improvements to overall comfort.

But it was the rise of the computer age and modern technology that really took the orthodontic treatments to the next level. Today continuing research and development is producing greater advancements in the latest techniques such as 3-D digital radiography and computer-assisted diagnosis and treatment appliances such as Invisalign®. Invisalign and similar devices created by other companies are custom-designed to straighten teeth using clear plastic aligners or retainers (they are clear and non-colored) and used to replace traditional braces. Making clear aligners even more unique, they are removable while eating or brushing.

Many people have seen the commercials or even celebrities who are wearing "something" on their teeth, but it's not obvious what is that device – and that is the beauty of the latest generation of orthodontic treatments. A mouth full of metal braces isn't always necessary or even the ideal solution, especially for adults who are not looking to appear young that "way" with old-fashioned braces, but want to simply look younger with a gorgeous smile. Clear aligners are also ideal for image-conscious teens who would otherwise resist braces for social reasons. Sometimes it requires careful examination to even recognize the aligners are in the mouth.

WHO ARE ORTHODONTISTS?

So who are these men and women who decide to specialize in straightening teeth as their careers? Let's start with the basic description of what an orthodontist does per the website MyMajors.com. "Examine, diagnose, and treat dental malocclusions and oral-cavity anomalies. Design and fabricate appliances to realign teeth and jaws to produce and maintain normal function and to improve appearance."

That is what an orthodontist does, but what are the top knowledge and skills an orthodontist must possess? On that same website MyMajors.com it lists among the top three areas of knowledge to include medicine and dentistry and techniques to "diagnose and treat human injuries, diseases and deformities." The other two areas include abilities to manage customer and personal service followed by knowledge and skills in biology and proficiency in English language.

Orthodontists are typically creative thinkers who have an aptitude for both the sciences and the arts. They love to solve problems, and derive a genuine satisfaction from helping others. When applicants to orthodontic residency are asked why they want to be an orthodontist, it is not uncommon for them to answer, "Because I like to work with my hands and help people."

What kind of education is required to become an orthodontist? The road to becoming an orthodontist is a long and challenging one. After graduation from college, all dental specialists including orthodontists must first attend and graduate near the top of their classes from an accredited four-year dental school. After successful completion of dental school, the new dentist must then apply for acceptance to an accredited orthodontic post-doctoral program. These programs are highly selective, and only a small fraction of applicants get accepted.

In Dr. Glaser's case (he authored this chapter), he was one of only eight students accepted to The Boston University Goldman School of Graduate Dentistry out of over 400 applicants! Once accepted, the orthodontic student must complete a rigorous two- to three-year full-time training program including classroom and seminar work, direct patient care in the clinic, as well as complete an in-depth research project. Upon graduation, the student is presented with either a Certificate in Advanced Graduate Studies (C.A.G.S), a

Master's degree or Doctoral PhD depending on the program.

While any dentist may perform orthodontic treatment, only an orthodontist who has the years of required training and experience might call themselves a "specialist". In addition to the educational training, experience is important as well. Like any healing art, with the passage of time, orthodontists become "seasoned". Not only do they gain valuable experience treating their patients, it is incumbent upon the orthodontist to continue their education by attending classes and seminars to stay current with the latest developments in the profession.

Professional affiliations such as membership in the American Dental Association and the American Association of Orthodontists indicate that the orthodontist is interested in staying up to date with new developments in the profession. Some orthodontists are also educators – teaching at a university or dental school or speaking at seminars. These doctors tend to be leaders in the profession dedicated to the advancement of orthodontics and to delivering the very best care to their patients.

ORTHODONTICS – MYTHS AND FACTS

Many people have misconceptions about what is or is not true about orthodontics, braces or aligners. Many "orthodontic myths" are based on what we saw as children or teenagers: orthodontics always result in a mouth full of metal brackets and wire. Some of these misconceptions are no longer the case. New methods and technologies have greatly revolutionized the process to the point where people may not even notice you're wearing braces.

So what is the reality of straightening your teeth using the current high-tech solutions? Let's start with the myths, which include:

- Orthodontists only treat children.
- Braces are unsightly (today's aligner technology is actually clear).
- Orthodontic treatment is painful (some technology is marginally uncomfortable).
- Orthodontists only treat complex cases.
- Orthodontics take too long.
- Orthodontics can damage teeth.
- Orthodontic treatment is expensive.

In order to dispel those myths, here are the facts of modern orthodontics:

- **Not just for kids and teens** – 20 percent of all orthodontic patients are adults.
- **Clear and invisible** – new orthodontic technologies like clear aligners or braces are no longer obvious. Clear braces and aligners, which are removable, make treatment far less noticeable. Now you can smile and the first thing people see are not necessarily your braces, and aligners sometimes can barely be seen at all.
- **Increased comfort** – now with miniature braces, light high-technology wires, and clear removable aligners, pain and discomfort are greatly reduced. This means taking over-the-counter pain killers (acetaminophen or ibuprofen) usually clear up marginal discomforts and make the whole process quite easy to experience.

- **No case is too difficult or too small** – most orthodontic malocclusion problems can be effectively treated, from the very simple to the complex. Even if you just want that one tooth straightened or both upper and lower teeth – a wide variety of issues may be addressed with proper treatment.
- **No longer two or even four years** – many adults who were treated with orthodontic solutions might recall it taking up to four years and maybe even two different sets of braces. While treatment times vary on a case-by-case basis, the average treatment time for all cases is about a year.
- **No cement and no concern** – forget the old band-and-cement method that could damage teeth. Modern braces and adhesives are safe for the teeth if well maintained by the patient.
- **Too expensive** – maybe the cost was too much money in years past; however, over the last 25 years the cost of braces has increased significantly less than the rate of inflation. Most orthodontists offer extended, flexible payment plans, and many insurance companies cover a portion of the orthodontic fee.

WHAT TO EXPECT DURING OFFICE VISITS

Unlike some modern professions where the computer enables people to virtually work together or from a home domicile, orthodontics remain tied to patients, and patient treatment needs to be in an orthodontist's office. Since patients must consistently visit that office and see the orthodontist and his or her staff, this makes the office experience a critical, welcoming part of the experience. Orthodontists are mindful of creating a positive environment for their patient's comfort.

A beautiful office environment says a great deal. Let's first look at the reception area (we'll call it that instead of "waiting room" since making patients "wait" doesn't seem appealing). Is it clean and neat? Are the furnishing up-to-date? Are the magazines current? Is there ample comfortable seating? A tastefully decorated, clean and neat reception area says, "We care about our patients."

What about the rest of the office? While office designs vary greatly from one place to another, there are common themes that convey the right message to the patient. Modern equipment, pleasant lighting, neatly organized work areas, or no unpleasant or "dental" odors. These things tell the patient that the doctor and staff have devoted a great deal of time, effort and money to creating an environment that will allow them to work at peak performance to deliver the best possible care.

The people who populate that office make an impact and difference, too. When patients visit the office, they are not just seeing the doctor. They interact with office staff right from the greeting from the receptionist to the examination by the doctor to the exit from the office. Every aspects of this experience should leave a positive, upbeat impression that speaks to their treatment and care.

An excellent staff begins at the top. The doctor needs to set the vision for his or her practice and hire and train staff that share in that vision. There must be excellent communication between doctor and staff, and there should be continuing education and training on a regular basis.

The entire office experience for most orthodontists

these days isn't quite what it used to be for their parents. New high-tech devices have automated the experience both from the office paperwork to the orthodontic process. Many offices process patients in the reception area and use automated systems that address everything from patient check-in to visit history and examination notes and information taken right from the exam chair. Parents will also find the methods to keep kids and teens entertained through personal entertainment systems, movies and games that go well beyond the typical board game of the past – think the latest interactive video games. In fact, some patients love visiting their orthodontists. Many offices create such an entertaining and exciting environment, a trip to the orthodontist is something patients look forward to doing.

WHY SEE AN ORTHODONTIST?

Most people think that the most common reason to get braces is either crooked teeth or buck teeth. Orthodontic issues encompass far more than those two problems. The following briefly describes the various orthodontic issues (this book will go more in-depth on these subjects in the other chapters).

- Overcrowding – crooked or overlapping teeth.
- Spacing – gaps between the teeth.
- Overbite or "buck teeth" – upper front teeth protrude.
- Deep bite – excessive overlap of front teeth.
- Open bite – the upper and lower front teeth do not touch.
- Crossbite – upper and lower teeth bite in reversed position.
- Gummy smile – excess gum tissue displayed upon full smile.
- Underbite – lower teeth and jaw jut out too far.

- Traumatic bite – teeth bite abnormally against each other causing abnormal wear, chipping or loosening of the teeth.
- Misalignment of the facial skeleton – orthodontists play an important role in multi-disciplinary management of developmental facial deformities.

Bad habits can also contribute to the corruption of teeth. Some of these habits include:

- **Thumb-sucking** – a behavior developed in babies and children and involves placing the thumb in the mouth for self-soothing and often prolonged durations of time. The results can produce distortion of the palate and teeth.

- **Nail biting** – another (often nervous habit produced from anxiety or apprehension) of chewing on fingernails using teeth. It is associated with bruxism (teeth clenching or grinding) that wears down the tooth enamel and is destructive to the mouth.

- **Tongue thrusting** – also called "reverse swallow" or "immature swallow" is another behavior deleterious to the mouth and teeth. It produces a number of different abnormalities as well as speech problems.

These though are habits and behaviors. Orthodontic treatments are required to fix genetic and craniofacial issues. Early intervention is critical especially in young children where orthodontic remedies can reduce the severity of developing problems and reposition teeth prior to other dental work.

When correcting craniofacial problems, orthodontics play an important part of overall team management (with dentists and doctors) of severe problems such as cleft palate, which is a congenital split of the roof of the mouth.

Additionally, orthodontic treatment and early intervention prevents self-esteem problems, especially in children where their self-image is beginning to form. Young children and even school-age children often have not learned to control what they say and do to others. As a young person's self-image develops, harmful teasing and comments about something a child cannot control can detrimentally impact that child sometimes for the rest of his or her life. Teasing and name-calling does hurt. While Bugs Bunny is a cute and adorable cartoon character, no child wants to be called "Bugs" or "buck-tooth beaver". This destructive impact can last a lifetime.

Further into adulthood, poor self-esteem and lack of self-confidence impacts personal and professional success. A man or woman who isn't self-confident or believes in his or her self-worth because of negative comments about her or her looks often feels bad inside and falsely believes he or she doesn't deserve better. While other societal and family behavior can also have a bad influence on behavior and lifestyle choices, poor self-confidence can lead to lack of romantic interests or selection of romantic partners who can be hurtful and cause further damage to the person's self-esteem. These situations often create a vicious cycle where the person continues to feel worthless or undeserving.

Professionally lack of self-confidence and self-esteem reduces overall success. For every person who feels a lack of confidence in the workplace, someone else might feel far more able to do a job and speak up and appear right for that position. It doesn't mean the person with the low self-confidence isn't indeed the better candidate. But outward perceptions and projection communicate the opposite message to superiors and decision-makers. Maybe the person with the image problem doesn't get hired at all or is continually passed up for promotion. His or her overall success in life is limited or reduced.

While getting one's teeth fixed doesn't guarantee inner transformation or promise to produce more dates or even promotions and success, it does promise a beautiful smile. As Dr. Glaser mentions in the introduction, a beautiful smile can transform a person's life and circumstances. Just look at the 40-year-old male who went from jobless and single to gainfully employed and involved in a relationship – all after finally having proper dental and orthodontic treatment.

Finally, the positive impact on overall health and wellness from straight teeth produces positive effects, too. Gum diseases resulting from crooked teeth such as periodontal disease arise from the inability to properly brush and floss teeth. Areas out of reach of the toothbrush or floss produce bacteria and plaque build-up. Left unchecked these problems produce everything from halitosis (bad breath) to gingivitis to tooth decay and rot. Studies (and you'll see information in later chapters) suggest connections to poor oral health is linked to heart attacks and incidences of cancer and other life-threatening illnesses. Gingivitis has been linked to premature and low-birth-weight babies in pregnancy.

Straight teeth are easier to brush and floss. Clean,

healthy teeth don't produce these oral diseases. Best news is of course teeth don't rot and fall out and cost tremendous amounts of money to repair or replace. While some people might have trouble with the costs of orthodontics, imagine the ongoing cost to your body and pocketbook to continuously repair damaged teeth. The overall benefits of orthodontic treatment outweigh the physical and monetary cost of repair and tooth replacement.

EVERY TOOTH PROBLEM HAS A SOLUTION

Today's modern orthodontics have a solution to every imaginable problem. Again, as you read this book you'll be reading in-depth about some of these procedures and solutions. Some of these modern treatments include:

- **Fixed braces** – either metal or clear braces bonded directly to the teeth. Kids love adding colors to their braces while adults prefer less-noticeable options like clear ceramic braces.
- **Removable appliances** – Orthodontists have a wide variety of removable appliances at their disposals to both straighten the teeth and keep them straight.
- **Functional appliances** – either fixed or removable devices that help to align the jaws and bite.
- **Invisalign®** – is clear, removable aligners that can straighten the teeth and align the bite without the need for fixed braces. This is a popular option for teens and adults.
- **Computer-assisted braces** – a digital scan of the teeth is obtained from which custom-designed wires are manufactured.

- **Self-ligating braces** – a metal arch wire clips into self-ligating braces allowing for improved control of tooth movement.
- **Accelerated orthodontics** – a recent development, there are several techniques that can be used to speed up tooth movement and shorten treatment time.
- **Temporary anchorage devices** or TADs for short – small screw-like devices that can enhance orthodontic treatment.

CASE STUDIES

The Dentist
Female Patient

SITUATION

Dr. A was an adult female patient who Dr. Glaser treated. She also happens to be a dentist. She presented to Dr. Glaser for treatment of a large space between her upper front teeth.

GOAL

She had the space her entire life and felt that as a cosmetic dentist she should have the best smile possible.

OUTCOME

She was successfully treated with Invisalign and has gone on to having a very successful practice. The increased self-confidence she gained helped her to become more comfortable speaking to her patients about the benefits of a great smile and healthy mouth.

The Executive Male Patient

SITUATION

Mr. B was an adult male patient with a high-powered executive position with a well-known international company. His teeth, however, had suffered from years of neglect. Several back teeth had already been extracted due to gum disease and decay, and his upper front teeth had loosened and flared forward. Mr. B realized that his unhealthy and unsightly smile were both an esthetic issue as well as affecting his overall health.

GOAL

Dr. Glaser teamed up with Mr. B's general dentist, an oral surgeon and periodontist to develop a comprehensive treatment plan to control the active disease in his mouth as well as reconstruct his bite and smile.

OUTCOME

After several years of extensive treatment—including Invisalign to reposition the flared upper front teeth, extensive gum treatments, and dental implants to replace the missing teeth, Mr. B's teeth and bite have been restored to a state of health and he can once again smile with confidence!

The Dancer
Female Teen Patient

SITUATION

Ms. C was a 16-year-old female patient who presented to Dr. Glaser as a very unhappy patient. She had seen three other orthodontists who all agreed that her large overbite could only be corrected with conventional braces. Ms. C was a dancer in her junior year of high school who aspired to someday be a choreographer. She could not imagine performing with braces, and absolutely did not want braces for her senior pictures or the prom.

GOAL

Dr. Glaser devised a treatment plan to correct Ms. C's overbite with Invisalign. He counseled the patient that if she was cooperative with treatment and faithfully followed all of Dr. Glaser's directions, she could be successfully treated without having to wear metal braces.

OUTCOME

After two years of treatment Ms. C, who turned out to be a delightful patient, was successfully treated with Invisalign. She has an absolutely beautiful smile and is now studying dance in college.

MUCH MORE THAN STRAIGHT TEETH

Orthodontic treatment is much more than just straight teeth and a beautiful smile. It's also improved self-esteem and self-confidence. In addition, orthodontic treatment creates healthy bites, which in turn leads to decreased tooth wear, increased longevity of the teeth, healthier gums and improved speech.

An orthodontist has years and years of special training and has devoted his or her career to helping his or her patients achieve a beautiful smile and healthy bite. Simultaneously scientist and artist, the orthodontist understands the complex biological processes involved in straightening teeth as well as the esthetic nuances necessary to achieve optimal esthetics. The orthodontist is often a therapist as well, skilled in dealing with the fearful child, self-conscious adolescent or the anxious adult.

When one makes the investment in having orthodontic treatment, he or she should feel reassured that he or she is placing himself or herself in the hands of a highly skilled professional devoted to the health and well-being of his or her patients.

"A smile is the light in the window of your face that tells people you're at home."

Author Unknown

CHAPTER 2
THE BEST AGE TO HAVE AN EVALUATION AND WHY
MAMNOON A. SIDDIQUI, DDS, MS

"An ounce of prevention is worth a pound of cure."
Benjamin Franklin

Following a philosophy to treat every patient with the best possible outcome and with high standards of care in a friendly and caring environment is what patients who visit Dr. Mamnoon A. Siddiqui's orthodontic practice can expect. He believes that in order to accomplish those goals, he needs the entire orthodontic team to be committed to constantly learning and upgrading their knowledge base to deliver the best experience to patients.

This belief system is reflected in his background, education and experience. Dr. Siddiqui was born and raised in India and moved to the Metro Detroit area of Michigan with his parents when he was just 12-years old. After graduation from Harry S. Truman High School in Taylor, MI, Dr. Siddiqui attended the University of Michigan – Dearborn for his undergraduate studies and earned his bachelor of sciences degree in biochemistry. He then attended the prestigious University of Michigan – Ann Arbor School of Dentistry where he earned a doctor of dental surgery and graduated among the top in his class. After dental school, he practiced general dentistry for a year before pursuing his orthodontic training.

After finishing dental school, he practiced general dentistry for a year before starting the orthodontic residency program at the University of Detroit Mercy School of Dentistry. While he was in the third and fourth years of dental school, Dr. Siddiqui wanted to gain some real-life experience in dentistry, and so he assisted local dentists at every opportunity.

While doing that, he met a couple of local orthodontists who encouraged him to pursue orthodontics. It was through his experience in assisting others that he found the orthodontic specialty very appealing and decided to pursue it as a career.

What attracted him most about orthodontics was the ability of the orthodontist to help transform a growing child's smile and confidence and possibly his or her outlook on life. His practice sees adolescent patients during a critical part of their growth when a child goes from being just a child to a teenager and young adulthood. This gives the orthodontist an opportunity to play an important part in their formative years when confidence and self-esteem are critical parts of their personal growth.

The orthodontist is the team's key leader and has to be the one who sets the standards in studying and evaluating key new technologies and techniques as they become available. He or she incorporates it into their practices for a better patient experience and treatment outcome.

Dr. Siddiqui's patients and their families today are savvy consumers in the digital age. Massive amounts of information that was once difficult or challenging to find is available at the tap of a finger. This same information can often be overwhelming and confusing at times. Consumers need an authoritative figure who can educate them about their specific conditions and give them confidence as to what will help them achieve their best smiles, best dental health, and overall dental success.

BEST AGE TO HAVE AN EVALUATION

Dr. Siddiqui's philosophy on the best age to have an orthodontic evaluation is simple. The best time to have an orthodontic evaluation is when parents notice something that they feel is not right with their child's teeth or when a child turns seven-years old – whichever occurs first.

Dr. Siddiqui has to separate the concept of "best time" for an orthodontic evaluation versus the "best time to start" orthodontic treatment. He always tells his patients, "We can't turn back the clock. If everything appears to be within a reasonable normal range we can place the child on recall for future evaluation and/or treatment."

He wants parents to understand that there are some situations that may best be addressed at an earlier stage in development while other conditions could be handled best later on when there is more growth and development. This is where the orthodontist's role as a trusted adviser and provider of orthodontic care becomes vital to the successful outcome of the child's orthodontic needs.

WHAT IS THE RIGHT AGE FOR THAT FIRST EVALUATION?

There is no actual right or wrong or perfect age for an orthodontic evaluation. The orthodontic profession, just like any other profession, has quite a varied opinion on this question. Many dentists and orthodontists have their own philosophy based on their knowledge and experience, and it can fluctuate based on trends in the profession.

The American Association of Orthodontists (AAO), the world's oldest and largest dental specialty organization, recommends that all children get a check-up with an orthodontist at the first recognition of the existence of an orthodontic problem, but no later than age seven.

The AAO's recommendation of an orthodontic evaluation by age seven is based on the fact that generally by this age most children have already erupted their first permanent molars and some anterior permanent teeth. With those teeth present, the orthodontist has sufficient information that can allow an assessment of the patient for different types of malocclusions and subtle problems with jaw growth amidst front-to-back and side-to-side tooth relationships.

At this early age there are many things that the patient's primary dentist or even their parents should look for that may benefit from an early orthodontic intervention. Most children will need only to be monitored and not treated until most or all of the permanent teeth are in place. Some conditions to watch out for are:

- Protruding upper front teeth (likely to be involved in trauma if left untreated)
- Underbite (lower teeth in front of upper teeth, can be a problem of jaw growth)
- Crossbites of any kind in the front or back (top tooth trapped behind lowers)
- Moderate to severe crowding (possible need for extractions)
- Early loss/extraction of baby tooth (will cause lack of space for permanent tooth)
- Ectopically erupting teeth (teeth growing in the wrong place)
- Extended thumb- or finger-sucking habit (try to quit by ages five to six)
- Missing permanent teeth or extra teeth (early planning to address consequences)
- Impacted teeth (teeth that are coming in the wrong place or direction)
- Ankylosed teeth (teeth fused to a jaw bone, may need to be extracted)
- Unusual tooth wear (especially in permanent teeth)
- Tongue thrusting (abnormal swallowing with tongue pushing the front teeth out)

Early detection and addressing some of the above-mentioned conditions will help in planning out the overall strategy for the individual child. It will also determine the most appropriate time for starting orthodontic treatment. One can never underestimate the psychological and social benefits of having normal-looking teeth even at an early age. Dr. Siddiqui has found that on many occasions he recommended waiting on a certain condition for further growth and development, but the parent/patient insisted on early treatment. They felt it would benefit their child socially or psychologically.

THE EVALUATION PROCESS

The orthodontic process over the years has been constantly evolving to make the patient more comfortable and feel at ease with all the different aspects of treatment. When a child visits the orthodontist office for the first time, they'll likely enter a warm, inviting, kid-friendly reception area that may even have some video games, iPads, or their favorite movies playing. The child may be able to work on some puzzles while they wait to be called back into the exam room to see the orthodontist.

Often times some parents already have gone through the orthodontic process when they were teenagers. They remember how things were back then, and they can relate to how things have changed for the better.

At Dr. Siddiqui's office they have a friendly front desk where staff greet the patient, and they check-in patients by using the iPad. A treatment coordinator will then walk the child back to the examination room and explain exactly what will be done that day to the patient and the parent's level of participation.

The treatment coordinator will generally take photos of the patient's teeth to see how they fit and also take photos of his or her face. Once this process has been done the orthodontist will come over and clinically examine the patient to make an assessment of his or her present conditions.

Sometimes a panoramic radiograph (a panoramic scanning dental X-ray is done of the upper and lower jaw. It shows a two-dimensional view of a half-circle from ear to ear. It is also taken to study the teeth that can't be seen in the mouth. The orthodontist will then show both the patient and parents on a large computer screen the child's teeth and how their conditions compare to a normal condition for a child at the same or similar level of development.

Any abnormal findings are thoroughly explained and possible solutions are discussed. Showing the clinical photos of the child's teeth is a great way to educate the child and parents about the present condition. Once they can see it with their own eyes they can begin to understand how the present condition is affecting their child, the child's growth and development, and how correcting it will improve or benefit their child.

The orthodontist looks for how the teeth and jaws deviate at this point from normal. The doctor determines whether this anomaly is something that can be treated later or will it significantly benefit from orthodontic intervention now. Most of the time, the evaluation at this age serves as a starting point in establishing a child's relationship with the orthodontist and his or her staff.

If during the initial visit, the orthodontist has determined that the child's present condition warrants further evaluation later on down the road or that a need exists to wait for eruption of more permanent teeth and/or growth, then the child will be placed on a recall, which is typically six months or a year. Just having this visit at an early age allows parents to ask questions and feel comfort in the fact that their child's condition is manageable.

MAKING IT EASY TO UNDERSTAND

Dr. Siddiqui believes that the most effective way for a parent to understand his or her child's condition is when the parent can see it for him- or herself in the photos that a treatment coordinator has taken. Once parent education takes place, then the orthodontist can get buy-in as to why it's important to treat now or why it may be prudent to wait until further conditions are met in the mouth.

Sometimes it is necessary to take a panoramic X-ray of the patient's teeth that goes around his or her head. This helps to visualize all the teeth that are present in the mouth and all the teeth that will erupt in the future. This is a great way to show all the teeth that are present and what factors will affect their eruption normally into the mouth.

Often the orthodontist will also make molds of the teeth to demonstrate the present condition. Technological advances now allow orthodontists to skip the traditional molds – digital intraoral scanners have gained wide acceptance and popularity. This technology also greatly helps the orthodontist to communicate clinical findings to the family and eases their understanding of the problems.

TREATMENT OPTIONS

After the evaluation, consultation and determination of the orthodontic status of the child, the orthodontist will likely place the child under one of the three categories:

A. Present condition will significantly benefit from orthodontic intervention now and active treatment is recommended now.

B. Present condition will benefit from early intervention, but certain conditions and/or teeth need to be present or erupted before initiating orthodontic treatment and the patient is placed on a recall for follow-up.

C. Present condition doesn't require any immediate orthodontic intervention but needs to be monitored closely for further eruption of more permanent teeth and growth/development to occur, and the patient is placed on a long-term recall for growth monitoring.

Early treatment options can vary greatly from simple counseling to something much more involved like an expander, headgear, facemask, braces, retainers, appliances for tongue thrusting or jaw correction, space maintainer, or a combination of any of the above. Some of these situations could be handled at the general dentist office or a pediatric dentist office while others will need to be done by the orthodontic specialist.

Each child is evaluated, and based on the findings of their individual clinical conditions a specific treatment plan is recommended for that child to maximize the benefits of the treatment. This will vary greatly from individual to individual since it's customized to the needs of a particular child. There's no cookbook or a one-size-fits-all strategy. One patient may benefit from early treatment while most others could be monitored until the rest of their permanent teeth grow in.

Some of the most commonly used appliances for early

orthodontic treatment in addition to limited braces are listed below (this is just a short list, an individual orthodontist may use a different set of appliances based on his or her knowledge or experience):

Rapid Palatal Expander – a palatal expander (also known as a rapid palatal expander), rapid maxillary expansion appliance, palate expander, orthodontic expander, Haas or Hyrax, is used to widen the upper jaw so that the bottom and upper teeth will fit together better. Use of a palatal expander is most often followed by braces to straighten out all the teeth now that room has been created.

Headgear – the most common treatment headgear is used to correct front-to-back discrepancies of the jaws. The headgear attaches to the braces via metal hooks or a facebow. Straps or a head-cap anchor the headgear to the back of the head or neck. In some situations, both are used. Elastic bands are used to apply pressure to the bow or hooks. Its purpose is to slow or stop the upper jaw from growing, thereby preventing or correcting an overbite.

The headgear can also be used to make more space for teeth to come in. In this instance the headgear is attached to the molars via molar headgear bands and tubes and helps to draw these molars backward in the mouth, opening up space for the front teeth to be moved back using braces and bands.

Protraction Facemask – reverse facemask or reverse-pull headgear is an orthodontic appliance typically used in growing patients to correct *underbites* (technically termed *Class-III orthodontic problems*) by pulling forward and assisting the growth of the upper jaw, allowing it to *catch up* to the size of the lower jaw. Facemasks or reverse-pull headgear needs to be worn between 12 to 22 hours per day, but typically 14 to 16 hours a day is effective in correcting the underbite. Overall wear time is usually anywhere from 12 to 18 months depending on the severity of the bite and how much a patient's jaws and bones are growing over this time.

Habit Appliance (to control thumb sucking or tongue thrusting) – like many potentially harmful behavior patterns, thumb sucking can be a difficult habit to break. Through the years, parents have tried a variety of home remedies, such as having the child wear gloves or coating the digits with a bitter-tasting substance — and even reasoning with their toddlers. Sometimes it works — but in other cases, the allure of thumb sucking proves very difficult to control.

If your child has a thumb- or finger-sucking habit that has persisted past the age of three, and you've been unable to tame it, then it may be time for you to visit the orthodontist. The orthodontist may consider treating your child with a "habit appliance" such as a fixed palatal crib or removable device. This crib isn't for sleeping — it's a small metal appliance worn inside the mouth and attached to the upper teeth.

How does it work? The semicircular wires of a palatal crib keep the thumb or finger from touching the gums behind the front teeth. Simply preventing this contact seems to take all the enjoyment away from the thumb-sucking habit — and without that pleasurable feedback, a child has no reason to continue the behavior.

Functional Appliances – a functional appliance is an appliance that produces all or part of its effect by altering the position of the mandible/maxilla. Also known as "dentofacial orthopaedic" appliances, these appliances utilize the muscle action of the patient to produce orthodontic or orthopaedic forces. These appliances work by posturing the lower jaw forward. These appliances are used while the patient is still growing, and the timing is dependent on the pre-pubertal growth spurt. These appliances may be fixed or removable. Some examples are listed below.

- **Herbst Appliance** — An Herbst Appliance corrects overbite by holding the lower jaw in a protrusive position. The Herbst Appliance is very effective in correcting large overbites due to small lower jaws in patients who are growing. These appliances can be fixed or removable.

- **Twin-Block appliance** — Twin-Block appliance removable appliance, and its high comfort level allows you to wear it 24 hours a day. This appliance actually is made up of two separate appliances that work together as one. The upper plate includes an optional expansion screw to widen your upper arch, if needed, as well as pads to cover your molars. The lower plate includes pads to cover your lower bicuspids. These two appliances interlock at an angle, and they move your lower jaw forward and lock it into the ideal position when you bite together. This new position, while temporary, will eventually become the permanent corrected position.

- **Bionator** — Bionators initially look like a sort of combined upper and lower Hawley retainer, but do not fasten to the teeth and are not used for post-brace removal treatment. Bionators are held in the mouth within the space that the teeth surround when biting. They are used to expand the palate and create space for incoming teeth.

- **Frankel appliance** – The Frankel appliance is a functional orthopedic appliance that is used to help create additional space for permanent teeth to erupt by expanding the arches. It stimulates growth of the lower jaw, which will better align the upper and lower teeth. The Frankel can also be used to help with protrusion or overjet by retracting the upper teeth and creating a better bite. Frankel appliances are typically worn full-time for 18 to 24 months and possibly longer if the permanent teeth have not fully erupted.

BENEFITS OF EARLY-AGE EVALUATION

For those patients who have clear indications for early orthodontic intervention, the benefits of successful outcome include:

- Proper guidance of the growth of the jaw.
- Proper regulation of the width of the upper and lower dental arches which support the teeth.
- Guidance of incoming permanent teeth into more desirable positions.
- Reduction of the risk of trauma (accidents) to protruded front teeth.
- Correction and/or elimination of harmful oral habits such as thumb or finger sucking or mouth breathing.
- Reduction or elimination of abnormal swallowing (tongue

thrusting) or speech problems.

- Improvement of personal appearance and/or self-esteem.
- Potentially simplifying and/or shortening treatment time later for comprehensive orthodontics.
- Possible reduction in likelihood of impacted permanent teeth.
- Preserving or gaining space for permanent teeth that may not otherwise come in or come in the wrong place.
- Establishing a working relationship with the child to help emphasize the importance of proper oral hygiene.

In addition to all the esthetic and functional benefits of early orthodontic intervention, we have to consider possible emotional, social and psychological benefits of the treatment as well. As mentioned earlier, some children are very conscious about how their teeth look. Some are even teased about it in school and elsewhere. And it all begins early when a child has their front teeth growing which usually happens around age six or seven.

By evaluating a child at the age of seven, we may be able to help the child feel more confident and better about their smiles, especially in such delicate and formative years of their lives.

ADVICE

In real estate, "location" is everything. Likewise in orthodontics Dr. Siddiqui likes to say "timing" is everything. Because each child differs in both physiological development and treatment needs, the orthodontist's goal is to provide each patient with the most appropriate treatment at the most appropriate time and in order to accomplish those goals, orthodontists have to be able to evaluate a child at around age seven or earlier if necessary. By doing this, parents will be giving their child the best opportunity for a healthy, beautiful smile.

Today most orthodontists offer a free no-obligation examination appointment. Dr. Siddiqui advises parents to take advantage of this opportunity. When you notice something or your dentist brings up something about your child's teeth or bite, take your child to the experts in malocclusion. The orthodontists are the professionals who have the training, knowledge and experience to be able to guide your child's teeth and bite into proper function and esthetics.

When you do visit the orthodontist, ask questions, such as:

- Why should this treatment start now?
- If treatment is not started now then what are the possible consequences? Can it wait? If it can, how long should we wait?
- How is the correction going to maintain?
- Is there going to be more work needed later?
- How is the treatment going to affect the child or his or her speech?
- And of course, the cost! Most parents are very concerned about paying for treatment "twice". They need to understand that this isn't paying for the same thing.

The point is, your orthodontist will be able to educate the child and parents on the child's currently existing conditions and demonstrate the benefits of treatment that the doctor recommends now. The orthodontist can discuss the potential consequences that may happen from not acting on the orthodontist's recommendation. Parents really need to understand what needs to be done and why. This can only happen if the orthodontist and their staff take the time to thoroughly explain everything. They can demonstrate by using terminology that the child and parents can understand.

One other thing to point out is these evaluations are best done in the presence of both parents. Some of the information presented or the aids used to present them is/are missing when discussed with the other parent – and this can lead to confusion.

So the bottom line is, Dr. Siddiqui strongly recommends to any parent who is concerned about their child's teeth or bite, they need to get the process started early. Parents should take advantage of the complimentary orthodontic evaluation that most orthodontists offer today and make the visit when their child turns seven or sooner if they notice something with the child's teeth that causes a concern.

Evaluation now can set the stage for successful treatment outcomes with healthy teeth and bite and a beautiful smile. One last thing to mention is that children at an earlier age (seven- to 10-years old) tend to be much more cooperative in following the directions and wearing of appliances than later on. Success of many of the treatment modalities is dependant on patient cooperation.

CASE STUDIES

CASE #1
Thumb-Sucking Girl

SITUATION

Seven-year-old girl, sucking thumb, parent has tried all the home remedies to get her to quit without much success. Patient has a significant anterior open bite as a result of the thumb sucking. Patient seems motivated to quit.

EVALUATION

Did the exam, showed the patient how the thumb-sucking is affecting her teeth and bite on the computer. Also showed the habit appliance we may need to use if her thumb sucking persisted. Patient was already motivated, we gave her a deadline, and counseled her on not just why it is important to quit, but also how and what the alternatives are if her thumb sucking persisted.

OUTCOME

She came back in six months. She was so excited to come to this visit. She had some good news for us, she had completely quit her thumb sucking. When Dr. Siddiqui examined her, her front teeth were already starting to come together! No actual treatment was done, just some counseling, education and motivation for the patient to quit thumb sucking, which if it had continued would have made her teeth stick out more and her bite would remain open.

CASE STUDY #2

Boy – Jaw and Teeth Issue

SITUATION

A six-year-old boy – parents and the dentist were concerned that the upper front teeth were behind the lower front teeth. Upon examination we noted that his lower jaw was sliding forward to make his lower front teeth slide in front of the uppers.

EVALUATION

We showed the patient and parents how this was affecting the gums of his lower front teeth and his upper jaw growth was being restricted. We made a recommendation to intervene now with a retainer that would have a ramp to guide the upper front to slide forward and over the lower front teeth. We instructed the patient to wear that retainer full-time and come back in a month.

OUTCOME

The patient did an excellent job wearing the retainer, and in just a month his upper front teeth were now in front of the lower front teeth.

CASE STUDY #3
Boy – Protruded Upper Teeth

SITUATION

An eight-year-old boy who had very protruded upper teeth, which had already been chipped a couple of times.

EVALUATION

We showed the patient and the parent how the protruded teeth were so susceptible to trauma. We recommended orthodontic intervention now to reduce the upper-teeth protrusion. In this situation we placed some braces and wires and retracted those upper front teeth.

OUTCOME

His teeth were now retracted. Braces were removed, and the patient wears a retainer at nights. We placed him on recall for more comprehensive orthodontic treatment when all the permanent teeth erupt.

CASE STUDY #4
Girl – Crowded Teeth

SITUATION

Another eight-year-old female patient, who lost a primary tooth too early, and the parents waited too long to have the space maintainer placed. This caused the other teeth around that space to move and take up the space that was necessary for the permanent tooth to erupt there. If nothing was done now, things would continue to get worse.

EVALUATION

A simple orthodontic intervention was recommended now to regain the space and maintain it until the permanent tooth erupted there. This situation involved placement of braces on the teeth in the affected arch, using some springs to regain the space and maintaining the space until the permanent tooth erupted.

OUTCOME

Waiting in this situation may have lead to lack of space for proper eruption of the permanent tooth and possible extraction (s) later. Now space is available for the tooth to come in.

CASE STUDY #5
Boy – Face and Jaw Development

SITUATION
An eight-year-old male child, who had a very narrow upper jaw and his upper front teeth were behind the lower front teeth. His upper face was underdeveloped and lower jaw was ahead of the upper jaw.

EVALUATION
We showed his condition to him and his parents. We recommended early treatment now to help correct his condition now while his jaw bones are still immature. In this case, we recommended a palatal expander to widen the upper jaw followed by a protraction facemask for 12 to 16 hours a day to help pull the upper jaw forward with elastics. We also used some braces on the upper front teeth to properly align the upper teeth ahead of the lower teeth.

OUTCOME
This worked really well as the child was very cooperative and his jaw bones were immature enough to respond well to the orthopedic/orthodontic forces.

As all the above cases illustrate, a proper early evaluation with an orthodontist set the stage for a successful outcome with healthy teeth and bite and a beautiful smile.

CHAPTER 3
SELF-LIGATING BRACES
DR. ALEXA A. ALBORZI

Dr. Alexa Alborzi lives her life with the maxim of "*Do onto others as you want done to you*." This has found its way into her career as well. Even when she chooses treatment modalities, she considers, "Do 'I' want that done to me?"

Dr. Alborzi started her career in orthodontics 21-years ago. As the phrase goes "time sure does fly when you're having fun." She feels that way about her work – and she really means it. She couldn't have chosen a more fulfilling and fun career.

Her career began with her specialty education at the University of Connecticut Health Center. Her training was with the use of twin brackets (AKA standard braces) with a heavy emphasis on biomechanics. This was fortunate because it gave her a very strong mechanical background for solving problems. She also taught twin bracket biomechanics for 14 years as an adjunct professor at the University of California, San Francisco Orthodontic Department.

With the biomechanical orthodontic education and her unstoppable thirst for more knowledge, every year she has taken 50-plus hours of continuing education to build on top of her formal training. The first 10 years, she practiced using the standard twin brackets and all the auxiliary appliances that are needed in conjunction with braces to accomplish the treatment outcomes desired.

It was the delightful few days she spent at Dr. Damon's (the creator of Damon Braces) office that changed her career from there on. She felt re-energized and very excited to deliver a type of treatment to her patients that could be effective, comfortable, faster, and consistently produce superior outcomes. Even better was that all those qualities allowed her to treat her patients with the same philosophy she had been treating them with before.

Her philosophy has been to create beautiful, natural, wide smiles and balanced faces without extraction, if at all possible. What was so refreshing was that she could do away with all the "torture" devices that she routinely used in the past. She tossed them all out the window! Those torture devices included: Palatal expanders, lingual arches, headgears, lip-bumpers and molar-distalizers (devices that push teeth in the back of the mouth further back).

She spent three days at Dr. Damon's office for training on this new technique, which is formally called self-ligating braces. Some may think braces are braces. That is true to some extent, but unique qualities of self-ligating braces require a completely different viewpoint on treatment and treatment planning. Treatments which without a doubt would need extractions or surgery no longer require that. That planning would require some additional knowledge and forethought with this system of braces. She has heard or seen many orthodontists complain about or fail at using self-ligating braces – they use them as if the braces are just another bracket (brace). Training and additional courses that she has taken are essential to successfully using this system.

So that's the story of how Dr. Alborzi fell in love with self-ligating brackets!

MALOCCLUSION – AND WHY TREAT IT?

Perfect teeth are straight, fit together perfectly, and don't overlap. Unfortunately, only 30 percent of the population enjoys this type of bite.

Malocclusion is defined as improper fitting of the teeth together. Teeth can fit poorly in many dimensions: front-to-back or side-to-side. They can be crowded. They can protrude and retrude or have no overlap. All these malocclusions have names. Here are the definitions.

Different types of malocclusion are classified as follows:

1. **Class I** is actually when the bite fits properly front-to-back, however if teeth are crowded or spaced, it is considered a Class I malocclusion.
2. **Class II** is when upper teeth are positioned ahead of the bottom teeth.
3. **Class III** is when bottom teeth are positioned ahead of the upper teeth.

All these classes of malocclusion can have additional problems such as crowding, open bite, deep bite, protrusion etc.

Open bite is when the top teeth don't overlap the bottom teeth, when you have this problem it is hard to get the lettuce out of your sandwich. Individuals who have this problem usually demonstrate excessive wear on their back teeth. Back teeth suffer fractures and end up needing crowns.

Deep bite is when the top and bottom teeth overlap too much. Individuals who have this problem usually demonstrate excessive wear of their front teeth, and this is visible as shortening of teeth.

The above classification is a brief overview of problems which may exist in your mouth. There are a myriad of things that may present in the mouth that may additionally complicate a bite. Periodontal problems, jaw-growth discrepancies, cross-bites, and tooth-size variations are a few of these problems.

You may ask, why does a malocclusion (bite problem) require orthodontic treatment?

If you have a normal bite, teeth "interdigitate" (which means the teeth interlock like the fingers of two clasped hands) properly during function. This proper function reduces untoward forces on the teeth which cause poor wear, fractures, gum recession, and even gum disease caused by heavy forces.

Here are some potential issues due to malocclusion:

CROWDING: Plaque and tartar buildup harbor harmful periodontal bacteria that increase risk of periodontal disease (gum disease), tooth and bone loss.

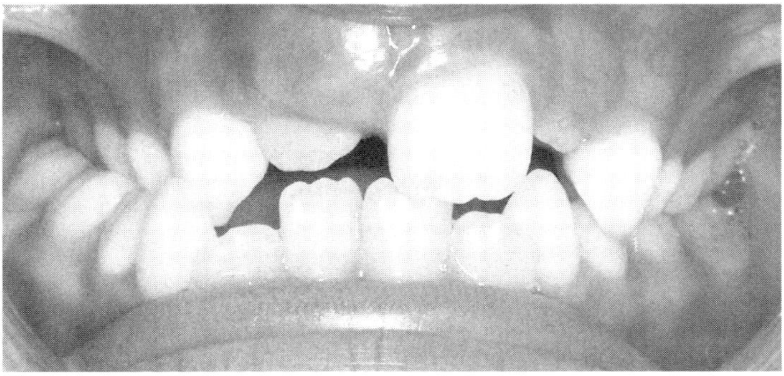

SPACING: Food lodges between your teeth, which causes sore, tender gums and increases risk of periodontal disease.

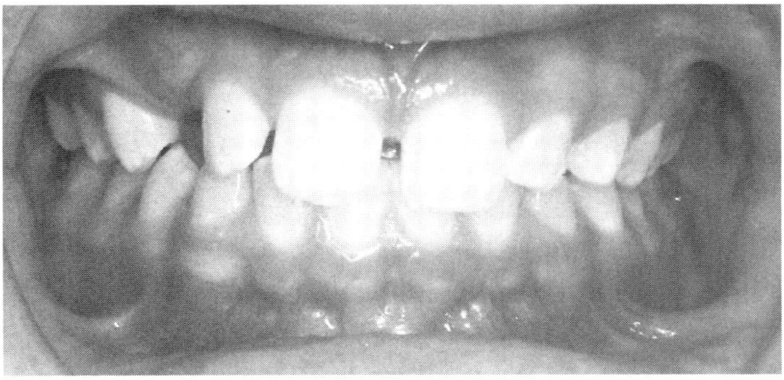

DEEP BITE: Lower teeth over-erupt and can damage the palate. This leads to premature wear and chipping of the front teeth.

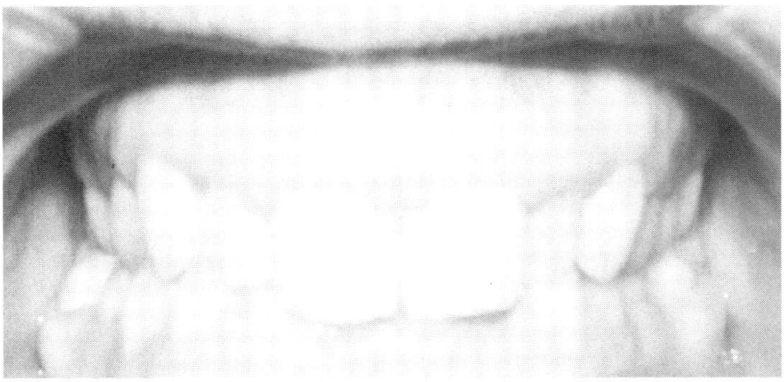

CROSS-BITE: Premature tooth wear and risk of chipped teeth. It can cause abfraction, which is a small notch in the tooth at the gum line. Due to untoward forces on the teeth, periodontal disease, tooth, and bone loss may occur.

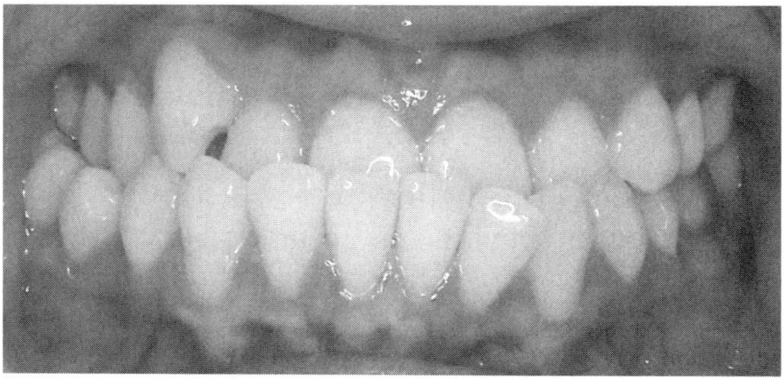

EXCESSIVE OVERJET: Chipped or fractured front teeth during function. It can increase chance of trauma to front teeth that may even cause tooth loss.

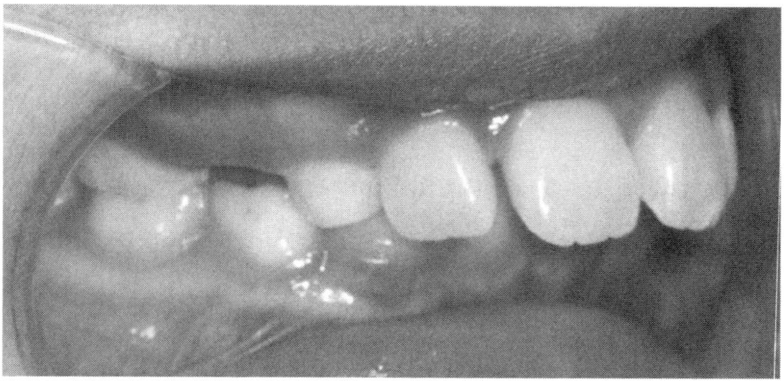

EDGE-TO EDGE BITE: Increased risk of teeth chipping and breaking, jaw-joint pain, chipped and worn-down front teeth.

OPEN BITE: Abfraction, which is a small notch in the tooth at the gum line. Gum recession, loose teeth, and bone loss can occur. Excessive, premature wear on back teeth is seen.

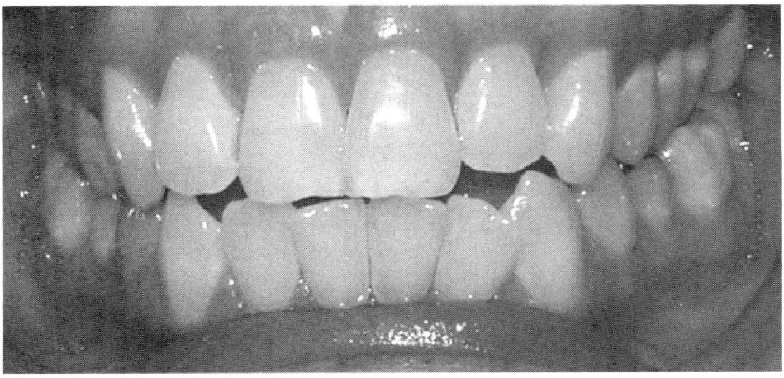

Has Dr. Alborzi given you enough reasons to straighten your teeth?

Malocclusion is a potential health risk. If left untreated, malocclusion can lead to periodontal disease. Periodontal disease has been found to increase risk of atherosclerotic cardiovascular disease (hardening of the arteries).

In addition, malocclusion causes premature wear of teeth, and over time this can worsen and even result in tooth loss.

SELF-LIGATING VS. OTHER TECHNIQUES

You as a consumer may think braces are braces! They are those metal or clear things put on teeth to make teeth straight.

Not all braces or techniques in orthodontics are the same. They practically all have advantages and disadvantages over each other. When an orthodontist gets trained, he or she may be trained in one technique or multiple techniques during his or her residency programs. Most of us as we practice we find what works best for us and matches our vision of how we would like our patients to be treated and what their treatment outcomes will be.

Types of Braces:

1. Metal Braces / Traditional Braces

When one mentions braces, usually this is the type of braces that come to mind. You see them as just plain silver or decorated with colorful rubber ties. They are also called twin brackets because they have two wings and the rubber tie holds the wire in place and allows the wire to move the tooth.

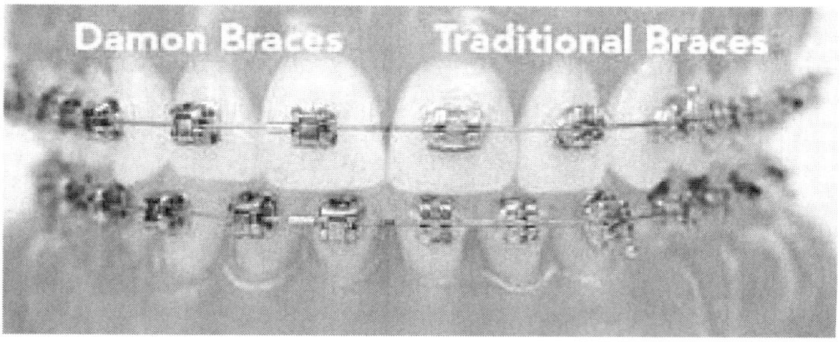

2. Clear / Ceramic Braces

This is the same as the above metal braces, except that they are clear and better for those who do not wish to advertise their braces very loudly! Most adults choose this type as it is less conspicuous. They tend to be bulkier than metal braces as it is a more fragile material therefore the additional bulk adds to its strength.

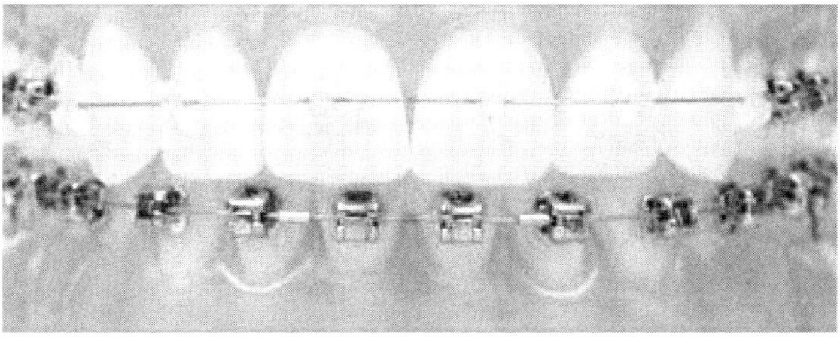

3. Self-Ligating Braces
This type of braces are designed as if there is a tube to put the wire through. However, instead of rubber bands to hold the wire in place, an adjustable gate allows wire to be held in place. This adjustable gate is the key to many advantages this type of brace has.

4. Lingual Braces
Lingual braces are totally invisible, unless you open your mouth real big. The braces are placed on the back of the teeth instead of the front. It is quite technique-sensitive and is not very commonly used. They can be irritating to the tongue, and they have many limitations.

WHY RECOMMEND SELF-LIGATING BRACES OVER OTHER TYPES?

Because of the unique qualities of this type of braces, Dr. Alborzi can treat patients more often without extractions, surgeries, and additional unwanted and invasive appliances. But more importantly, she can create amazing smiles which cannot be created without extractions. She likes to know that the faces of her patients stay young as long as possible, and she didn't cause their faces to age faster. She loves to see her patients go through the experience of treatment without much discomfort or too much investment of time out of their busy lives.

Dr. Alborzi personally uses a type of self-ligating braces called Damon Braces. It was Dr. Damon who actually put the word self-ligating back into use by his pursuit of excellence in this type of treatment mechanism. The type of self-ligating brace that Dr. Alborzi uses is called passive self-ligating, which compared to the active self-ligating has a spring that is activated and pushes on the wire – and that spring increases the pressure on the wire.

The main difference between all these types of braces is the amount of force they put on the tooth. The passive self-ligating braces generate 600x less force compared to traditional braces. The active self-ligating braces generate 300x less force. The lower force allows the blood vessels around the teeth to not get shut off and therefore a more healthy process of bone turnover occurs.

The lower the forces, the healthier the bone turnover, and therefore teeth typically move much faster and gentler. Lighter forces allow the bone to be oxygenated by blood vessels around the teeth – this helps the teeth and bone move together where we didn't believe they could move. It also reduces the damage to the roots of the teeth (AKA root resorption).

The questions are:
Would I want to have root resorption?
Would I want to experience 10x more discomfort?

Would I want to go to the orthodontist every four to six weeks?
Would I want to look older 20 years down the line because I had teeth pulled?
Would I want to have extra pieces of metal in my mouth?
Would I want to wear headgear?
Would I want to have four teeth pulled?
Would I want to have surgery if I didn't have to?

Dr. Alborzi's answer to all-of-the-above questions is a resounding NO!

It is true that sometimes she still has to recommend surgery or extraction of teeth. When she plans and diagnoses treatment for her patients, she has their facial esthetics in mind as well as a beautiful smile.

There are times that if she makes adequate room for all the teeth (which she is able to do most of the time), the facial balance of the patient will be poorly effected. Therefore, the facial beauty and harmony is the determining factor on these more extreme options of treatment – extraction and surgery.

AMAZING EXPERIENCES AND OUTCOMES

When Dr. Alborzi trained and started practicing orthodontics, the only tool she had was the standard twin braces with the beautiful color ties!

She had resorted to accepting that type of brace as the way to treat patients and even taught it to her students for 10 years. After all, she was trained at the University of Connecticut, and they were the experts in bio-mechanics. She could move teeth anywhere – and she really could.

Moving teeth was not any problem. However, she was

not happy with what it took to get her patients the amazing outcomes that she wanted them to have. The missing ingredient was their experiences while going through treatment with respect to discomfort, not having to extract their teeth, facial harmony, and time out of their lives.

In 2002, she started using the Damon System. A new era of orthodontics had begun for Dr. Alborzi. She didn't have to put her patients through unnecessary discomfort associated with high forces, uncomfortable auxiliary appliances like headgear, and she could achieve amazing and consistent results. Patients no longer had to routinely get expanders or extractions of teeth. Surgery was not the only option for some of them. She was elated and remained that way.

Additionally, she found her patients, many of them who were adults, too busy with work and family. School-age kids didn't want to miss so much time out of school, or the schools didn't want them out for appointments. Being part of an athletic team made it even more difficult for kids to come to their visits every four to six weeks, as their coaches wouldn't allow that absence. Good news is with the self-ligating braces, patients don't have to come to the office more than every eight to 10 weeks at a time.

Today, we all face even more challenges with time! Dr. Alborzi overcame all the challenges relate to time by using the self-ligating system. At their first appointment, patients will get all of their braces and without any need to come in a week prior to get separators to make room for rings (bands) on their teeth. Everything gets bonded to teeth, simply and comfortably. Then patients return 10 weeks later.

It happened that as Dr. Alborzi wrote this chapter, she consulted with a young patient who was told he needed expanders, and a myriad of other treatments. She told the parents that how she was going to treat their son might sound very simplistic compared to what they had heard so far. However, that is the beauty of what she can do with the Damon braces – she can give their son a great outcome without putting him through unnecessary discomfort and procedures.

She should also mention here that she has never received any calls from anyone complaining about a discomfort that they can't handle – this is not an exaggeration! This situation is quite different from most of her experiences with standard braces.

SELF-LIGATING BRACES: FROM THE FIRST TO THE LAST APPOINTMENT

First Appointment

When you arrive for your first appointment, the most important information is your chief complaint. Dr. Alborzi likes to know what is not optimal and what is really concerning you. She makes sure she addresses this concern.

At the initial appointment, she likes to take a panoramic radiograph. In a child, this X-ray shows the general pattern of dental development, where the developing permanent teeth are located, and how they are erupting. Teeth can develop in unusual locations and grow in unintended directions compared to normal growth. A panoramic X-ray can also show if there is adequate space for all permanent teeth waiting to erupt.

In an adult, a panoramic X-ray, shows the level of bone around the teeth, the roots of the teeth, and areas of the jaw beyond the roots. She additionally evaluates the shape of the Temporo-mandibular Jaw Joint (TMJ) for any anomalies. It is important to see a big picture of the jaws, since tooth movement is not limited to only moving the crowns of the teeth. We are moving the crown *and* roots. If this type of X-ray is not taken, there are occasionally pathologies that would be missed.

The next important diagnostic tool she uses are the photographs of the face. In addition to the photographs, she performs a thorough examination of the teeth and face.

All of the above data, allows Dr. Alborzi to make a final or preliminary diagnosis depending on the complexity of the problem. Additional records needed after the initial examination are a cephalometric X-ray, which is a measurement of the head, from a profile view and molds of the teeth. With the above data, she can determine your needs with respect to your chief complaint and her findings. Diagnosis is the same irrespective of what type of treatment modality. However, when it comes to the ability to achieve certain outcomes, it is important to use the right tool.

TREATMENT PLAN

Once she determines your needs by assessing all the diagnostic information then she sets out and plans your treatment steps. This step determines where your brackets should be placed, and even details what angulations (the action of making angular) within the bracket is needed to give you the fastest and best outcome. This is done with Dr. Alborzi in front of the computer and assessing all the gathered information. You can call it homework!

BONDING DAY

This is an exciting day for most patients. It is exciting for kids because they have always wanted braces. It is exciting for adults because they are finally doing what they had put off for a long time or they look forward to the day their braces will come off.

To place your braces your lips and cheeks must not touch the teeth. To do that we place a soft cheek retractor, and it makes your mouth look like a fish. Your teeth are then polished and prepared for bonding. Dr. Alborzi places a special sealant over your teeth to prevent cavities. Then the doctor places your braces using a direct technique of one by one. There is an indirect way of doing this in which the braces are first placed on a mold then delivered as a group onto your teeth. They both deliver the same outcome at the end. The bracket placement takes about 10 to 15 minutes. The cement that glues the braces to your teeth is cured with a blue light and then wires are placed.

The wires that are placed are space-age wires developed originally by NASA. They have a memory quality that prevents them from taking a permanent deformation (the action of changing shape or distorting, especially through pressure). This quality allows these wires to put the least amount of pressure on your teeth and keep doing that for 10 weeks. They are part and parcel to the delivery of low forces with self-ligating braces.

At this first appointment we sometimes may ask you to wear some rubber bands that hook your top teeth to the bottom teeth in certain patterns. These allow the teeth to move more in one segment than the other. For example, if the front teeth stick out too far, they can put more pressure on those front teeth and help them to retract to the ideal position.

Once the wires are placed, we give you instructions as to how to care for your braces and what to expect.

HOW TO TAKE CARE OF YOUR BRACES

At your initial appointment we will review general care for your braces.

- You will be given a list of hard foods to avoid or watch for.
- You will be instructed how to brush and floss.
- Various tools such as an inter-proximal toothbrush, dental wax, floss threader, etc., will be given to assist you in better care of your teeth.
- Brushing time has to increase to five minutes to really clean around the brackets, gum line, under the wires and tops and insides of the teeth.
- Flossing is more difficult, and a floss threader or something like *Supper Floss™* can be used.
- Dr. Alborzi also recommends water-picks such as the ones from Waterpik™ or Sonicare™.

Kids usually give up all together on flossing because it is much harder. Dr. Alborzi asks them to floss top teeth one night and bottom teeth the next night to make it more manageable.

THE FIRST WEEK

This is the week that everyone has to be patient in order to get used to their braces. New sensations are experienced in the mouth. The lips function against the braces and initially effect speech, and braces rub against cheeks.

Dr. Alborzi recommends salt-water rinses starting a week prior to placement of braces in order to toughen and make tissues of the mouth ready for this new experience. It definitely makes it easier.

If an area is getting sore due to too much rubbing, patients are given wax to cover up brackets or areas that rub.

The first week, she also suggests using a manual toothbrush as the mechanical ones won't feel very good against sensitive teeth.

The word "sore" just got mentioned? Yes, when teeth move, you will experience soreness of teeth when you try to eat, especially the first three days. Plan ahead and make shakes and soups the first three days. Some individuals may take up to five days, but that is rare.

This is where the self-ligating braces are amazing – there is so little discomfort. But if you've never had braces before it still is not be a lot of fun to have sore teeth. Most people don't need any medication to help with the discomfort they experience. Dr. Alborzi wore Damon braces about four years ago, and she can confidently confirm this.

ADJUSTMENT APPOINTMENTS

Every eight to 10 weeks you arrive for adjustments. The main purpose of an adjustment visit is to move teeth further toward their ideal position. The main procedure during adjustment is a wire change. As we make wires larger and stiffer, the brackets move the teeth to the expected position.

Adjustment appointments may also include changing of bracket position on a tooth. Sometimes teeth are so crooked that it is not possible to originally place brackets in the best position.

The adjustment appointment will again cause your teeth to get sore, sometimes not as much as the first appointment. You can use the bite wafer to chew on to help alleviate the discomfort more quickly. Devices like Acceledent™ that help speed treatment also reduce discomfort.

Most orthodontic treatments require elastic wear. These rubber bands provide additional directional pressure to help move teeth. At adjustment appointment, we check to see how you are doing with our instructions for elastic wear. Dr. Alborzi has to be honest: 80 percent of patients do not follow instructions as they are supposed to do. This only results in added cost and time to their treatments. Following elastic instructions well is the best way you can ensure timely removal of your braces.

You may need to come for a visit in-between your adjustment appointments. Usually these visits are due to teeth straightening and causing wires to poke out. Sometimes, eating foods that are a bit harder may cause a bracket to break off as well. Eating with braces is a bit different than without. It's best to eat smaller morsels of food and position the food more on the inside of the mouth versus in the cheek area. Big chunks of food between cheek and braces can generate enough force to break the brackets – after all our jaws can produce as high as 1,400 Newtons of bite force.

Working together as a team with the orthodontist is the sure way to complete your treatment in a timely manner. Keeping appointments is crucial as well. One missed appointment can set you back for weeks.

After all this a beautiful healthy smile awaits you!

A HEALTHY, BEAUTIFUL SMILE AWAITS YOU!

Anywhere from 10-28 months is the average time treatments may range. The day the braces are removed is the most joyous day, and we do celebrate it with you.

Removing braces is mostly mechanical. The braces get taken off by putting a certain pressure on them that causes deformation that pulls them off the glue. Once braces are off, there is residual glue on your teeth. The residual glue is polished off, leaving teeth smooth and beautiful.

Most individuals don't find this process uncomfortable. There are the rare few, especially those who always clench their teeth and already have sensitive teeth, who don't find this an easy process. However, we have our ways to make you as comfortable as possible.

If you have done a great job with your dental hygiene, your smile will look amazing right away. If your gums are swollen, it will take a few weeks before your smile becomes amazing. Dr. Alborzi recommends getting your cleaning and checkup after a month so your gums can improve, and the dentist can do a better job cleaning and examining your teeth.

When teeth have been crooked for a long time, there could have been poor wear patterns on the teeth, and straightening them is not enough to create a perfect smile. This is when additional dental restorations such as crowns and veneers maybe indicated (See below).

Before Braces

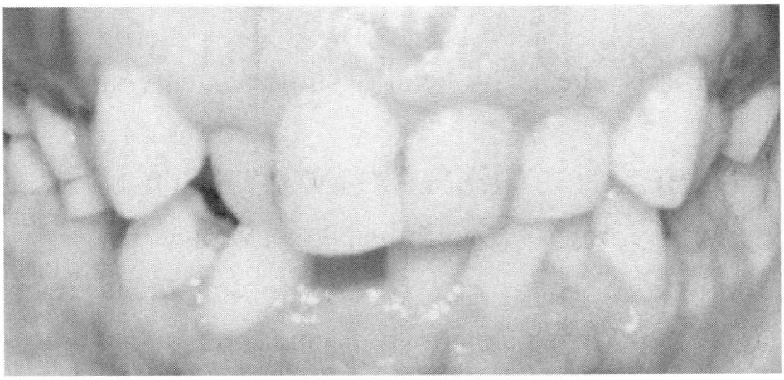

After Braces

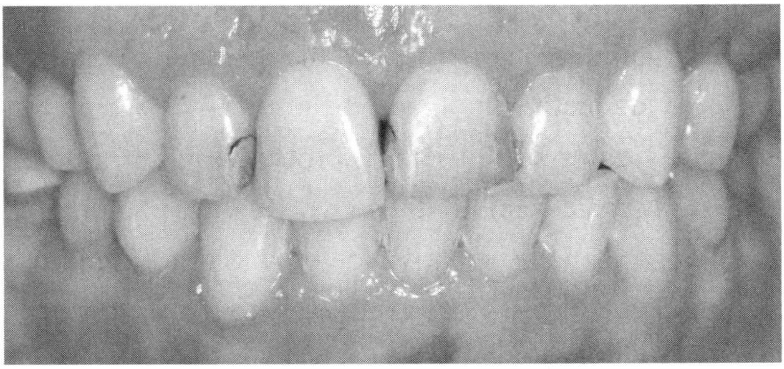

After Restoration

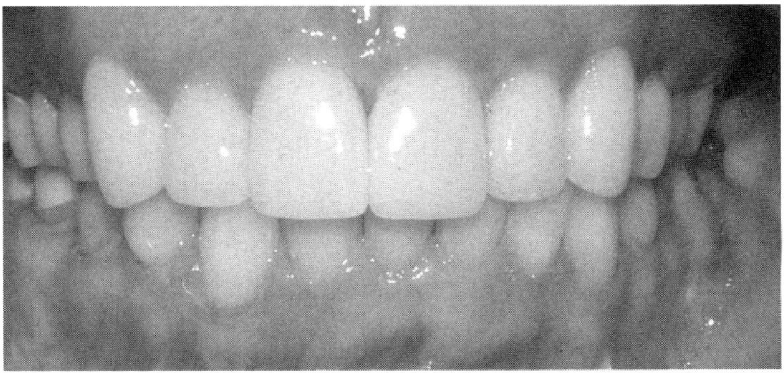

Other time, the gum coverage on the teeth has up and down levels or there is too much gum over the teeth hiding its full length. In these cases, we can do what is called a gingivectomy (trimming of gum), which uses a dental laser. This procedure is relatively simple. The level of discomfort may be as much as a pizza burn.

If you have missing teeth or restorations that need changing, now is the time. Implants (false teeth) are also placed when orthodontic treatment is complete.

Important Note: Never have a dental implant placed if you are considering orthodontic treatment. An implant is solidly fixed in the jaw bone and cannot be moved.

WHAT WILL KEEP YOUR TEETH STRAIGHT AFTER BRACES?

As our bodies are constantly changing, so will our teeth change as time passes. Teeth are constantly on the move because of muscles of the tongue and face and chewing forces. Teeth also have a tendency to move back toward their original positions.

Dr. Alborzi asks her patients, "If there was something that would keep their faces from getting old would they wear it every night?" The answer is a resounding yes.

Retainers are the devices that keep your teeth from "wrinkling". Once your braces are removed, new molds are taken and retainers will be made from them.

She recommends wearing retainers only at night time. Over the past 20 years, she has found that about eight hours is sufficient time to keep her patients' teeth straight, and about two percent will need to wear their retainers initially more than that.

Occasionally some teeth like to move during the day hours when the retainer is not worn. In those rare cases, we place a bonded retainer on the insides of the teeth to keep them fastened.

It is best to keep retainer wear as a part of your routine for life – that is, only if you'd like to keep your investment of a beautiful smile for a lifetime.

Just like shoes, retainers do wear out. Dr. Alborzi recommends a new set of retainers every two to five years, depending on how hard you are on them.

Retainers are made after the braces are removed or sometimes just one visit prior to removal. Molds (copies of your teeth) are taken or a digital scan can be done to create a copy of your teeth. From that copy retainers are made.

There are several types of retainers. There is the old-fashioned Hawley retainers that are a combination of wires and acrylic. This type of retainer works excellent as long as you are very good about wearing them. Once your teeth move, due to its rigidity, it doesn't easily push your teeth back to the original straight position. That's why Dr. Alborzi prefers the Essix type of retainers that look like an aligner. These hold your teeth straight really well but are more fragile and need to be replaced every two to five years. Another great thing about them is that they protect your teeth from bruxism (grinding of teeth during sleep).

Keep your investment by wearing your retainers!

Hawley Retainer

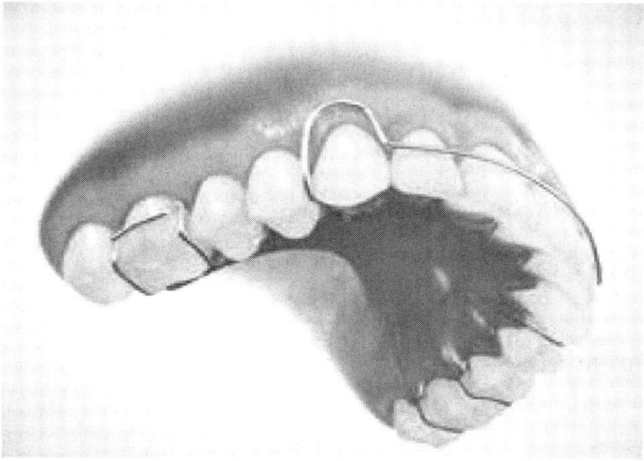

Clear Retainer

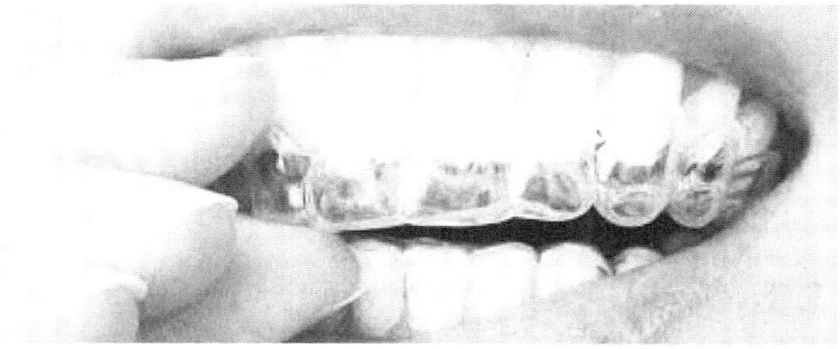

What do patients say about their experience:

MY TEETH ARE PERFECT!

"Before coming to Dr. Alborzi, I went to two other orthodontists. One told me she could not work on my teeth because my case was too 'complicated'. The other orthodontist told me if I wanted to have perfect teeth I would need jaw-surgery or if I opted not to do that I would need extractions but my overbite would never fully close.

"With Dr. Alborzi, I didn't need jaw surgery or extractions. And my teeth are perfect!

"I can't put into words how happy I am with my new smile! It truly has changed my life, and I feel like a new, more confident person.

"Dr. Alborzi uses the Damon System which allowed my teeth to become straight and perfect without surgery or extractions. The other orthodontists used older, traditional braces. I am so grateful to have found Dr. Alborzi. She and her entire staff have made a huge impact on my life. They are the nicest people and have treated me so well over the past two years of my treatment.

"So thank you Dr. Alborzi and every single person at Alborzi Orthodontics for giving me the opportunity to have a beautiful smile and the confidence I longed for! I didn't need jaw surgery or extractions. And my teeth are perfect!" — RR

THE DAMON BRACES WORKED PERFECTLY!

"My two daughters and I are all patients of Dr. Alborzi. We had heard great things about Damon Braces, and she was the only orthodontist in our area to use this most recent technology.

"After meeting with her, we were thrilled to find out that my daughter, who had a cross-bite, overbite and crooked teeth, would be able to go without the terrible metal expander in her palette. The Damon braces worked beautifully and she had a whole new smile in less than one year. It was easy and painless.

"The office staff is upbeat, friendly and very organized. The facility is extremely clean. We highly recommend Dr. Alborzi for your orthodontic needs." — KC

VERY PLEASED WITH THE RESULTS

"I have been very pleased with the results provided by Dr. Alborzi. She is a master of producing a wonderful arch form with the teeth nicely in alignment. She makes the smile fit the face.

"Other practitioners routinely leave anterior open bites in order to finish their cases earlier or do not include second molars, which come erupt and introduce occlusal disharmony. I believe that Dr. Alborzi routinely finishes cases as well as they can be done, and that is saying a lot." — RO, Local General Dentist

CHAPTER 4
EARLY INTERCEPTIVE TREATMENT/GROWTH AND DEVELOPMENT
DR. MARTA BAIRD

Collaboration and working with others is the central theme of Dr. Marta Baird's background in dentistry and orthodontics. She graduated from the University of the Pacific, Arthur A. Dugoni School of Dentistry in 2008, which was roughly six years ago from the first print edition of this book in early 2015. After graduation, she practiced general dentistry for one year with her mother, who is also a dentist. In the same timeframe, she taught dental students how to make crowns and veneers as well as how to perform local anesthesia on each other.

She used that year to grow as a professional and work on her master's degree research project with the orthodontic department. She also began a 27-month residency at the University of the Pacific. Over the next three years after graduation from orthodontic residency and completion of her clinical exams to become an American Board Certified Orthodontist, she joined three separate practices before opening her own private practice. Each of these practices gave her a unique private-practice experience.

One office, own by a prosthodontist who specialized in the complex restoration of multiple missing teeth with implants, enabled her to learn new skills. While she worked with this doctor once a week, she helped him prepare his adult patients for their restorations by creating the correct spacing for their dental implants. Whenever a tooth is lost, over time the other teeth space out and grow into the space. If a replacement is not made immediately, orthodontic treatment is necessary to restore the teeth to their initial positions.

The orthodontist she joined had been in practice for over 30 years, focusing on interceptive orthodontic treatment. At this office she had the opportunity to study several decades' worth of records. Patients who had been seen when they were eight-years-old, had been given treatment, and then had returned with their own children. One of the greatest lessons learned was not just what works, but what holds up over the long run. These parents had straight, beautiful teeth and now they wanted their children to have the same wonderful experiences.

Her early treatment method is based on her training in orthodontic residency as well as her experiences in private practice. Her love of collaboration also nurtured her learning experience and skills, as she has been taught from other orthodontists who have been in practice much longer. She enjoys learning about what has worked for other orthodontists. She likes to study available literature and understand what has been proven to be not only efficient, but also the best treatment for patients. She also focuses on another patient concern, which is to be cost-effective.

WHEN TO GO FOR EARLY TREATMENT

Every patient who comes to Dr. Baird's practice can expect a positive experience and treatment that results in a healthy, functioning bite. A functional smile (AKA functional occulusion) is a stable bite where there is no over- or underbite and the joints, muscles, teeth and ligaments structures line up. When a patient's bite is off one way or the other difficulties with chewing and even headaches can arise. The orthodontist's main goal is to solve those problems. The doctor also aims to create straight, white teeth that look great on the patient's face and create a beautiful smile.

Orthodontic problems are sometimes caused by genetics. These root causes include a small mouth, large teeth, or a slower-growing lower jaw, which can create an overbite. Environmental influences can be a cause as well and include: thumb-sucking habits that can cause bite problems; premature loss of baby teeth due to cavities; trauma that results in less space for permanent tooth eruption; or mouth breathing.

Why does early treatment make a difference? In many cases a patient waits until adolescence, which people commonly believe is the best time to start orthodontic work, when all permanent teeth have erupted. At this point, your orthodontist would be required to make compromises to straighten the teeth. The teeth don't necessarily fit well with the patient's face even though those teeth might appear straight in the mouth. Needless extractions are then done to correct overbites when growth modification from early treatment would have been a more ideal result.

When early treatment is done with a comprehensive

approach that addresses most or all aspects of the malocclusion, later treatment may either not be needed or will be limited to less then a year to correct minor cosmetic issues. A malocclusion is imperfect positioning of the teeth when the jaws are closed.

Early treatment corrects existing or developing skeletal and dental imbalances to improve the environment (in the mouth) before the eruption of permanent teeth is complete. By starting orthodontic treatment at a younger age (before all the baby teeth have fallen out), the overall need for complex orthodontic treatment involving permanent tooth extraction and orthognathic surgery is reduced. Orthognathic surgery is used to correct conditions of the jaw and face related to structure, growth, sleep apnea, TMJ disorders, malocclusion problems owing to skeletal disharmonies, or other orthodontic problems that cannot be easily treated with braces.

Early treatment may prevent more serious problems from developing and could make treatment at a later age shorter and less complicated or even eliminate future treatment. In some cases, the orthodontist will be able to achieve results that may not be possible once the face and jaws have finished growing. An early orthodontic evaluation gives children the best opportunity for a healthy, beautiful smile.

The goal is to provide each patient with the most appropriate treatment at the most appropriate time.

Early treatment provides a number of positive outcomes. It does the following:

- Guides jaw growth
- Lowers the risk of trauma to protruded front teeth
- Corrects harmful oral habits (e.g., thumb sucking)
- Improves appearance
- Guides permanent teeth into a more favorable position
- Improves the way lips meet
- Reduces the need for permanent tooth extractions and surgical treatment.

Initiating treatment in the mixed dentition does not imply that treatment will be provided continuously with braces from when the upper lateral incisors erupt to when the second molars are aligned (from ages seven to 12).

A concentrated period of early treatment is initiated in the mixed dentition and has a defined beginning and end. Following growth guidance, intermittent observation of the patient during the transition to permanent dentition is a major component of early treatment. In simple terms, the patient regularly comes in for follow-up office visits so the orthodontist can observe progress and ensure results of early treatment are not lost.

Early treatment improves facial balance and creates adequate space for permanent teeth to erupt so that permanent tooth extractions are not necessary.

EARLY TREATMENT – AGE SEVEN

A good age to evaluate a child's mouth are from ages seven to eight. Parents can help evaluate the situation by understanding what is normal in a seven-year-old child.

What is normal in a seven-year-old:

- The permanent first molars and incisors have erupted.
- The incisors (front teeth) are spaced.

After these teeth come in, there is a delay of two to three years before any further permanent teeth appear. This allows time for the orthodontist to make corrections and adequate space before more permanent teeth grow in.

What is NOT normal in a seven-year-old:

- Crossbite of front teeth – top teeth are behind bottom teeth
- Crossbite of back teeth – top teeth are inside the bottom teeth
- Crowding – overlapping of front teeth
- Open bite – front teeth do not meet when back teeth are closed
- Protrusion – front teeth stick out over the bottom teeth
- Deep bite – bottom teeth touch the roof of the mouth
- Underbite – the lower teeth sit in front of the upper teeth when the back teeth are closed
- Spacing – large gaps between the front teeth
- Oral habits – sucking on thumb, fingers

Other additional things NOT normal in a seven-year-old:

- Early or late loss of baby teeth
- Difficulty in chewing or biting
- Mouth breathing
- Jaws that shift or make sounds
- Speech difficulties
- Biting the cheek or the roof of the mouth
- Facial imbalance (chin to one side)

By ages eight to 10, the mid-face and lower jaw have only completed half of their total cumulative growth. That means there is still a significant amount of growth remaining for the orthodontist to use to correct a jaw-growth imbalance. The ability of the skeleton to respond positively to orthodontic treatment diminishes as maturation approaches. Without the room to grow to manipulate teeth versus extract them isn't desirable. It can be difficult to close gaps once the teeth are removed (in some cases) and make the teeth align.

Therefore, the ideal age to schedule an appointment for an orthodontic checkup is no later than age seven. Orthodontists can spot subtle problems with jaw growth and emerging teeth while some baby teeth are still present. While your child's teeth may appear to be straight, there could be a problem that only an orthodontist can detect.

A check-up may reveal that your child's bite is fine. Or, the orthodontist may identify a developing problem and recommend monitoring the child's growth and development. Then if indicated begin treatment at the appropriate time for the child. In other cases, the orthodontist might find a problem that can benefit from early treatment. Early treatment may prevent or intercept a more serious bite issue (that could require extraction of adult teeth or jaw surgery) from developing and may make treatment at a later age shorter and less complicated. In some cases, the orthodontist will be able to achieve results that may not be possible once the face and jaws have finished growing.

Early treatment may give your orthodontist the chance to:

- Guide jaw growth
- Lower the risk of trauma to protruded front teeth

- Correct harmful oral habits
- Improve appearance
- Guide permanent teeth into a more favorable position
- Create a more pleasing arrangement of teeth, lips and face

Again, the goal is to provide each patient with the most appropriate treatment at the most appropriate time.

WHAT TO EXPECT AT THAT FIRST VISIT

When a child comes in for the first time, it's important for him or her to feel comfortable with his/her orthodontist and the office and staff. Many children have seen braces before on their classmates or on older siblings. Your orthodontist discusses the fun aspects of braces such as the different color options for your braces. Then he/she discusses the details of treatment with the parents. Eye contact and reassurance are important to gain the patient's trust before any treatment begins. Dr. Baird and her team of qualified professionals want families to know they will be well taken care of, and that they will have a great experience along the way.

Today's modern technologies have changed the entire patient experience from the past when patients waited in quiet waiting rooms, went to their seats in the orthodontist chair, opened their mouths, and the doctor did his or her job. Now the office visit has transformed into an enjoyable, exciting experience.

Dr. Baird's practice in particular provides a "fun" office visit with video games, iPads and toys in the waiting room as well as movies to watch on movie glasses during long procedures, which are all part of creating a comfortable atmosphere for patients. Dr. Baird says she has even been told that younger siblings of patients have begged to be taken along to orthodontic appointments just to spend time in her office!

At the first consultation to determine if early treatment is needed, an examination of the teeth and X-rays (provided by the dentist) is preformed by the doctor. Occasionally an additional X-ray is needed to determine where the un-erupted permanent teeth are located in the jaw. This X-ray is often taken in the office on the same day if needed, and a copy is sent to the dentist for their records.

The exam takes into consideration:

- The main concern of the family or family's dentist.
- Pertinent medical/dental history – any past problems that might affect the treatment.
- Facial evaluation: How the teeth fit into the face, if they are too far forward or too far back in the face; how the teeth look when smiling; and how the lips come together with any asymmetries.
- Dental evaluation: How the teeth fit together when the child is biting, and if the face is symmetrical when the child bites (sometimes a child may bite so that her lower jaw goes to one side, this is called an asymmetry).
- Checking if there is any crowding. Which teeth have grown in, and if it is in the correct order (sometimes a baby tooth falls out too early and a tooth grows in before its turn. This can block other permanent teeth from growing in correctly).
- Discussion if the child has any habits such as teeth grinding or clenching, thumb or finger sucking, or breathing through

his/her mouth during sleep, and even chronic allergies.

- Periodontal evaluation: gingival health, oral hygiene.

Thumb Sucking Really DOES Hurt Teeth

Thumb sucking is a habit that frustrates parents of children probably more than any other habit. Among the parents' concerns are teasing by classmates or siblings, and its effects on speech and chewing ability.

Thumb sucking starts out as an instinct to help young children self-soothe. Thumb sucking under the age of five is not as much of a concern as thumb sucking once permanent teeth have begun to erupt. At age six the permanent molars first begin to grow in; their growth can be affected by a prolonged sucking habit.

The dental effects of thumb sucking are narrow arches that can result in posterior crossbites (upper teeth fit inside the lower teeth), crowding of the permanent teeth, and anterior open bite (top and bottom teeth don't touch).

To successfully stop the habit, the timing must be right. Usually treatment begins when the child is five years of age or older and wants to stop the habit. Family participation is critical to success. There are better times to intervene then others. Bad times, for example, might be during periods of stress, such as a move to a new home or school, the arrival of a new sibling, or changes in routines. These stresses are not conducive to successful intervention.

A book I recommend to parents to help them unite with their children to achieve a common goal titled *Helping the Thumb-Sucking Child* by Rosemarie A. Van Norman.

If a child is unable to stop the habit on his/her own, treatment may involve an appliance that fits across the roof of the mouth so that the thumb does not fit as comfortably as before. The habit usually stops immediately, and the appliance is left in place for three to six months to make sure it doesn't return once the appliance is removed.

It is critical that the child wants to stop the habit and that treatment is presented as an aid and not a punishment.

After evaluating and considering these various scenarios, the next steps involve taking records if more information is needed and if treatment is indicated. Photographs are also taken of the face in two positions – smiling and at rest. Also, photos are taken of the teeth from different angles.

Next is the modeling and scanning process. Different procedures are done. Among them are panoramic X-Rays (X-rays of upper and lower jaws that show two-dimensional views of the a half-circle from ear to ear). These X-rays show where the teeth, which have not grown in, are located in relation to the teeth that are present. Orthodontists can see the direction of how a tooth is growing. Dr. Baird can also detect if there are missing teeth or if a tooth needs more room to grow in properly.

Before treatment begins, the orthodontist and patient discuss goals of treatment and what will be accomplished within the timeframe. Discussion of habits come under focus. While thumb sucking (see sidebar) is among the top habits of concerns, other behaviors that impact the mouth and teeth come under consideration. Those practices include: sucking on the lower lip, which can cause the upper teeth to flare out more. Fixing an overbite, though, with orthodontics creates less room for the lip to fit between the teeth and therefore stops the habit.

Chronic mouth breathing can cause an anterior open bite in which the front teeth do not touch when the child bites on his/her back teeth. This can be caused by many things including chronic sinus infections or allergies and decreased nasal airway. When the mouth is open the tongue moves between the front teeth, resulting in the open bite. The first step in treatment of the open bite is to determine the cause of mouth breathing, so your orthodontist may need to work with your pediatrician. An expander can be used to increase the nasal airway as part of orthodontic treatment

---

EARLY TREATMENT OPTIONS

The ideal orthodontic solution intercepts a developing problem (malocclusion) before it can increase in severity. The solution corrects definitively, eliminating the need for additional extensive treatment. It should start and finish when children are in elementary or middle school. At this age, tissue adaptation and response is optimal, and children are enthusiastic about braces. This makes them more willing to cooperate with their treatments. The ideal solution should also minimize cost, treatment time, and the need for extraction of teeth.

There are three common approaches in orthodontics:

Minimal: This approach recommends using a comprehensive "one-phase" treatment once all the permanent teeth have erupted and all of the primary teeth have fallen out. Early treatment is avoided except for the correction of impacted molars or anterior and posterior crossbites. When early interception is required, treatment is nominal, and the remaining components of the malocclusion (e.g., overjet, overbite, open bite, etc.) are addressed in a second phase of treatment.

Generally orthodontists using this approach try to time the comprehensive treatment to coincide with the onset of the adolescent growth spurts (11- to 13-years old for girls and 12- to 14-years for boys). Permanent teeth are extracted to provide space to correct crowding and large overjets. This comprehensive orthodontic treatment usually takes two to four years, and it has several drawbacks:

- Increased severity – some forms of malocclusion worsen with age. For example, a mild to moderate overjet or crossbite can become more severe between the ages of seven and 11. In some instances, increased severity can cause a case that original only needed orthodontic treatment to now require orthognathic surgery (see early definition).
- Social aspects and patient cooperation – adolescent children are less enthusiastic about wearing braces and more reluctant to follow through with or cooperate with the needed treatment. Orthodontic treatment that coincides with this crucial age is more likely to involve compromises and less likely to achieve the desired results.
- Need for extraction – by the time eruption of the permanent teeth is complete, the hard and soft tissue components of the jaws are less adaptable. Orthodontic treatment that begins at such an age is more likely to involve extraction of the permanent bicuspids.
- Incidence of injuries – children with protrusive maxillary incisors are more prone to traumatic incisor fractures before adolescence.

Two Phase: As the name suggests, this approach involves two phases of treatment. Phase I usually involves orthopedic approaches to expand (RPE), retract (headgear), or protract (facemask) the maxilla. The objective is to limit the extent of treatment needed in Phase II.

Ideally Phase I lasts one to two years and is followed by a Phase II for one to two years once all the permanent teeth have erupted. The main issues with this approach are increased costs and longer treatment time because two phases of treatment are required.

Another issue is the lack of standard treatment protocol. A number of appliances can be used with this approach, and each can be manipulated in various ways.

Headgear: headgear attaches to the braces via metal hooks or a facebow. Straps or a head cap anchor the headgear to the back of the head or neck. In some situations, both are used. Elastic bands are used to apply pressure to the bow or hooks. Its purpose is to slow or stop the upper jaw from growing, thereby preventing or correcting an overjet.

Twin block – a removable plastic appliance that patients bite into to hold it in place in the mouth. It postures the lower jaw forward so that the overrate is corrected.

Herbst – similar to the twin block in that it holds the lower jaw forward during growth, but it is fixed in place as-is and is non-removable.

Then there are removable appliances that can perform minor tooth movement but depend on patient compliance and must be worn varying amounts throughout the day and at night

Expanders – expand the upper jaw to correct a narrow

upper jaw and allow the jaw to accommodate the upper teeth when there is not enough room

As a result, there is no consensus in treatment protocol available for orthodontists to follow. That means that Phase I can mean two very different things to two different orthodontists.

Interceptive Orthodontic Treatment: This approach leverages the biological and social advantages of the early mixed dentition (seven- to eight-years old), instead of waiting for the adolescent growth spurt.

It uses efficient mechanics to address most of the skeletal and dental components of a malocclusion during the early mixed dentition. It takes advantage of the more adaptive tissue response of the mixed-dentition growth period.

The key advantage of this interceptive approach is that it is comprehensive and addresses all components of the malocclusion. Treatment takes about two years, and the need for Phase II is eliminated in 90 percent of cases. For the 10 percent of cases in which Phase II is recommended, it involves a less complex, more cost-effective treatment that can be accomplished in less than a year. In addition to being cost-effective and time-efficient, this protocol eliminates the need to extract teeth by 99 percent.

Interceptive orthodontic treatment can be used to do the following.

Guide the growth of the jaws:

Class II – in this situation the upper teeth are too far forward in relation to the lower teeth. The lower jaw appears small and set back. If left untreated, this type of bite tends to worsen with time as pressure from the lower lip causes the upper teeth to move forward even more. Early treatment corrects the way the teeth fit together and the relationship of the upper and lower jaw.

Once corrected, the upper and lower jaw grow together in harmony to maintain the normal balance of the face. An upper jaw expander as well as braces can be helpful in treating this type of bite – it gives the lower jaw room to move forward.

Occasionally when the upper jaw has grown far ahead of the lower jaw, wearing headgear at night is necessary to hold the upper teeth and jaw from growing forward for a few months while the lower jaw catches up to correct the bite. It's important to time the correction so that the child still has a lot of growth left.

Without interceptive treatment, once the lower jaw growth slows down in teenagers depending on the severity, treatment may require removal of teeth, surgery, and three or more years of orthodontic treatment. Waiting for all of the permanent teeth may miss the significant growth opportunity, especially in early maturing girls.

Class III – when the lower teeth and jaw are ahead of the upper teeth, orthodontic treatment is needed to guide the upper jaw forward so that it is ahead of the lower jaw. In a normal bite, the upper front teeth fit just slightly forward compared to the lower teeth. At age seven to eight growth can be used to guide the upper jaw forward in the face.

When the upper jaw is small an expander is used to widen the jaw to the normal width along with a facemask. A facemask attaches to the teeth and pulls them forward using the forehead and chin as anchor points. Correction can happen in as little as six months in most cases.

This appliance is usually only recommended to be worn at home and to bed. The older the child (over age 10) the more rigid the upper jaw is to resist this type of correction. In this type of situation, if treatment is begun too late then the remaining options involve removal of teeth or jaw surgery.

Crossbite – in this type of bite, the upper jaw is narrow compared to the lower jaw. This means that there will be less space in the upper jaw for all of the permanent teeth to fit. Using an expander in a seven- to eight-year-old, which fits across the roof of the mouth to widen it, is relatively comfortable. Expanding at an older age such as 11 or 12 requires more pressure then at age seven or eight.

The expander may attach to the permanent teeth or to the primary teeth. It has a wire across the roof of the mouth to connect both sides. A small screw that can be turned in 0.25-mm increments, and it is used to gradually widen the upper jaw.

Improve the width of the upper and lower dental arches – sometimes children have narrow upper and lower dental arches. The shape that the upper teeth make can be a "V" instead of the ideal "U". Narrow arches result in less space for the permanent teeth. When left untreated, often the last teeth to grow in (the canines) simply do not have room. They may either not grow in at all (impacted) or will grow into the wrong place, which results in the appearance of "fang teeth".

Widening the upper jaw with an expander can create six millimeters of space for the permanent upper teeth and about five millimeters of space for the lower teeth. This is a significant amount of space since a moderate amount of crowding in a teenage patient with permanent teeth is four to six millimeters. Expansion creates room for the teeth before they have a chance to grow into the wrong place and gives room for the adult teeth.

Guide erupting permanent teeth to desirable positions – when an X-ray is taken at the initial exam and a permanent tooth appears to be growing in the wrong place, treatment may be necessary to prevent damage to the roots of the other permanent teeth nearby and to decrease the likelihood of the tooth becoming impacted (impacted teeth are those that should have come in but have not). Occasionally a permanent canine may grow more horizontally toward the roots of the front teeth rather than vertically into the mouth and into its correct position. Damage to the roots of the upper front teeth is irreversible and may cause those teeth to be lost.

Early intervention to create space for such a tooth and removal of a baby tooth to encourage the tooth to grow into the new space can save patients from more extensive and invasive treatment in the not-too-distant future. Waiting for all of the baby teeth to fall out in such a situation would be tragically too late. Not only does it pose a risk to the front teeth, but an impacted tooth would require surgery to remove the bone and gum covering it so that it could be brought into the mouth with braces.

In addition to permanent teeth that grow incorrectly due to genetics, a tooth can also grow incorrectly when a baby tooth is lost too soon. When a baby tooth is lost, the nearby teeth spread out into the space. One of the purposes of a baby tooth is to hold the space necessary for the permanent tooth until the tooth is ready to grow in and push out the primary tooth. When the baby tooth is lost too soon and the space closes, the permanent tooth no longer has a space reserved for itself. Without treatment the permanent tooth may be blocked from growing in or may grow in significantly out of place resulting in a longer treatment than if the space had been restored.

Lower the risk of traumatic injury to protruded upper teeth. When a child has front teeth that protrude significantly forward, these teeth are more at risk of trauma. After falling off a bike or being hit in the face with a ball, these teeth are the first to encounter the hard object or break the fall. This can result in knocking the teeth out and needing replacement teeth or breaking them to the point of needing extensive treatment to repair the damaged teeth. Early treatment can correct the position of protruded upper front teeth soon after they grow in. Waiting until all of the baby teeth have fallen out may be an additional four years in which these teeth could be susceptible to traumatic injury.

Help eliminate harmful oral habits such as thumb sucking or finger sucking which can cause open-bites (see sidebar above).

Reduce or eliminate abnormal swallowing or some speech problems. When the front teeth don't meet even when the child bites completely on the back teeth, this is known as an open bite. Having an open bite means that the tongue must come forward in-between the teeth during swallowing in order to create a seal or vacuum in the mouth. This abnormal swallowing perpetuates the open bite. An open bite can also result in speech problems for the same reasons. The longer the swallowing pattern or habit persists, the more difficult it is to break. Early treatment aims to close the open bite so that the tongue can rest against the roof of the mouth during swallowing instead of between the teeth.

Potentially simplify and/or shorten treatment time for later treatment if needed. When early treatment addresses all aspects of the malocclusion such as the bite and creating adequate space for the permanent teeth, only minor if any treatment is needed once the permanent teeth have erupted.

Often times the orthodontist will continue to monitor the eruption of the permanent teeth after the braces are removed. A retainer may be used to help guide the permanent teeth into place to avoid further treatment. If treatment is needed, it is usually less invasive than if early treatment had not been done. There will be fewer incidents of extractions, and the results will be more stable. When additional treatment is needed, it can often be accomplished with more esthetic and comfortable appliances such as Invisalign®. While not every teenager may be a candidate for Invisalign, early treatment exponentially increases their chances of being able to approach their treatment and use this modern technology.

CONCLUSION

Interceptive orthodontic treatment can have immense benefits to patients by preventing more serious bite problems and crowding from developing. In many cases, the orthodontist will be able to achieve results that may not be possible once all the permanent teeth have erupted because the face and jaws have finished growing.

Not every patient who comes in to see the orthodontist

at age seven will need orthodontic treatment, but the orthodontist specializes in evaluating each child so that they have the best opportunity for a healthy and beautiful smile and that each child is provided with the most appropriate treatment at the most appropriate time.

CASE STUDIES – EARLY TREATMENT

Clara, age 8

SITUATION

Clara has spacing between her upper and lower front teeth. Her back and front teeth fit together normally. Clara's X-rays show that all of her teeth are developing normally.

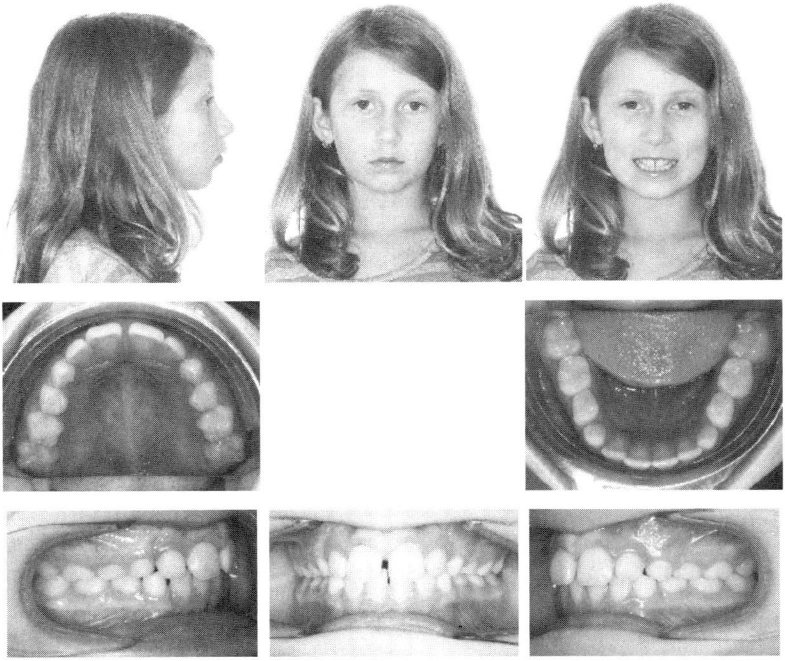

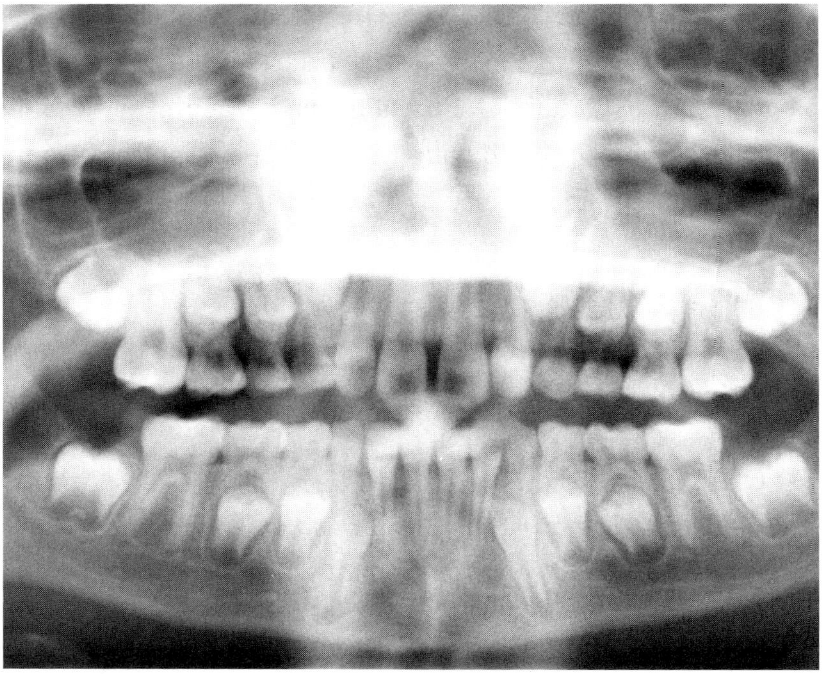

SOLUTION

Dr. Baird recommended that Clara wait until all of her permanent teeth come in to see if she would need any orthodontic treatment. The transition from baby teeth to permanent teeth uses up space.

OUTCOME

In Clara's situation, most of her spaces will be closed as the adult teeth grow in. She may not need any orthodontic treatment in the future.

Case Study 2
Louis, age 10 years old but his dental age is closer to 9.

SITUATION

He has four upper and lower permanent front teeth and four permanent molars, one in each quadrant. The rest of his teeth are baby teeth and are not loose. Louis is an excellent candidate for interceptive treatment because he has a deep bite, not enough room for his teeth, and his upper jaw is narrow (especially on the right where he has a crossbite).

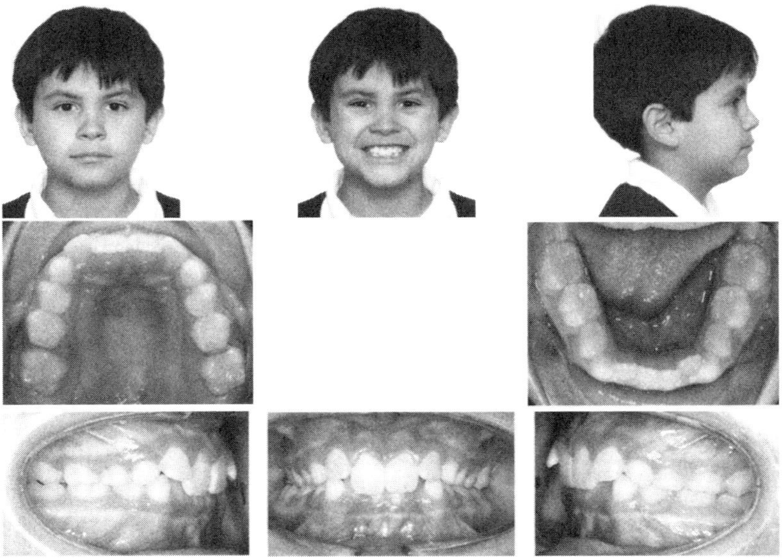

SOLUTION

Louis' treatment involved an expander and braces to create room for all of his permanent teeth as well as to fix his bite.

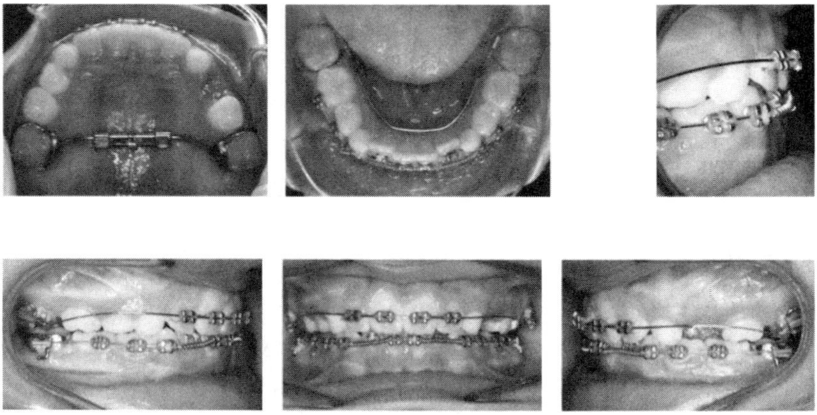

After 10 months of treatment we began to see more space in his upper and lower jaw. We began to see more of his lower teeth as his deep bite was corrected. His upper jaw was much wider to accommodate his permanent teeth.

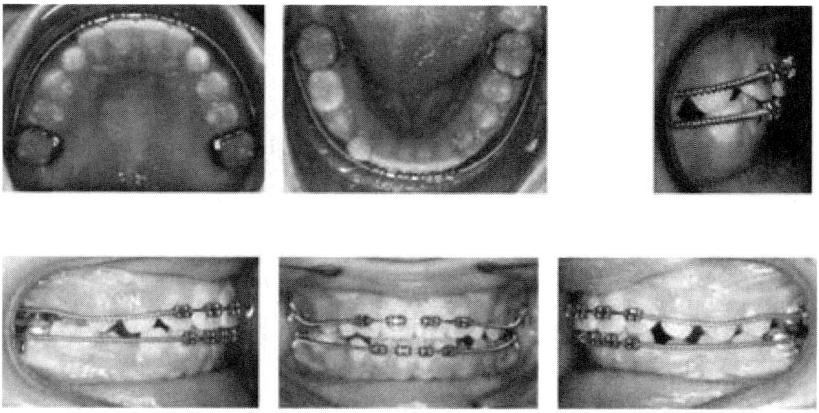

After 20 months we began to see the result of his treatment as more and more baby teeth fell out during treatment. By this time Louis was almost 12-years old since we began treatment later then the typical interceptive orthodontic patient (age eight).

OUTCOME

After two years of orthodontic treatment, Louis has entered his supervision/retention phase. He has an upper removable retainer that will be used to maintain the position of the adult teeth that have already grown in and also to coach the remaining permanent teeth into their correct position. On the lower arch he has a permanent retainer that will be replaced with a removable retainer once his adult teeth have completely grown in. Louis has a nice result with a good overbite and overjet. As his face continues to grow and lengthen and the adult teeth grow in, his upper front teeth will be tipped inward for a more upright appearance. In the meantime, their position allows room for the permanent canine teeth to erupt.

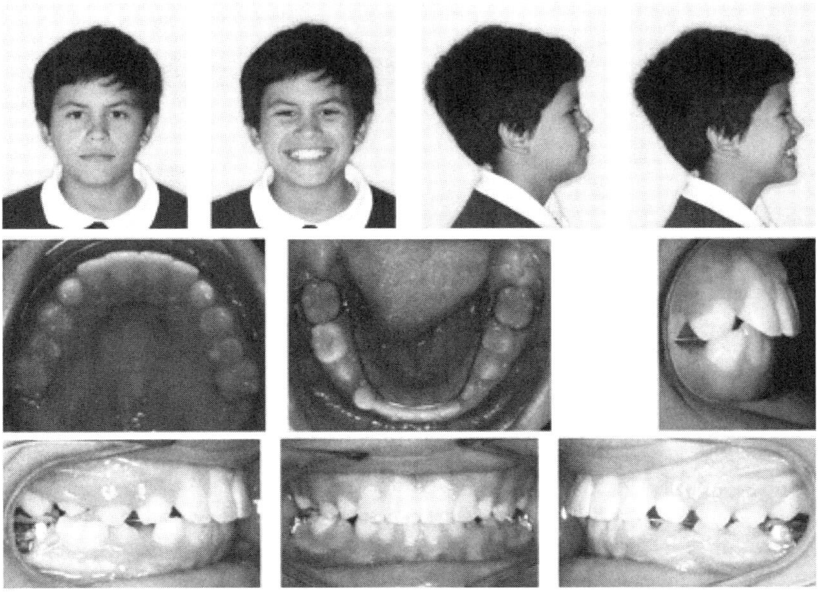

What is remarkable in Louis' case is the progress made with expansion of his upper jaw with regard to his upper left canine (upper right on the X-ray, third from the upper middle). This tooth was growing horizontally and toward the root of the lateral incisor. With expansion and arch development, this tooth changed its growth direction in order to move into the ideal position.

Initial X-ray

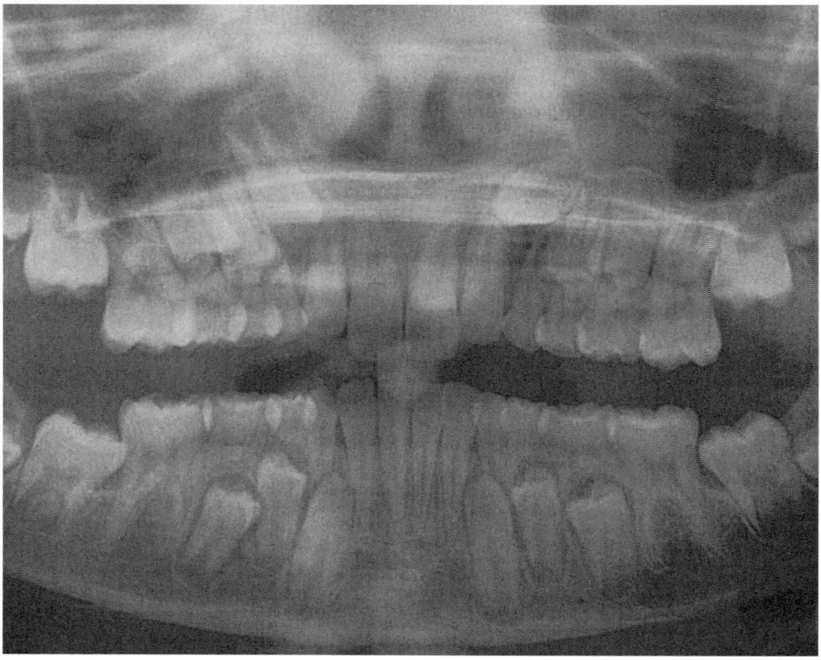

Final X-ray

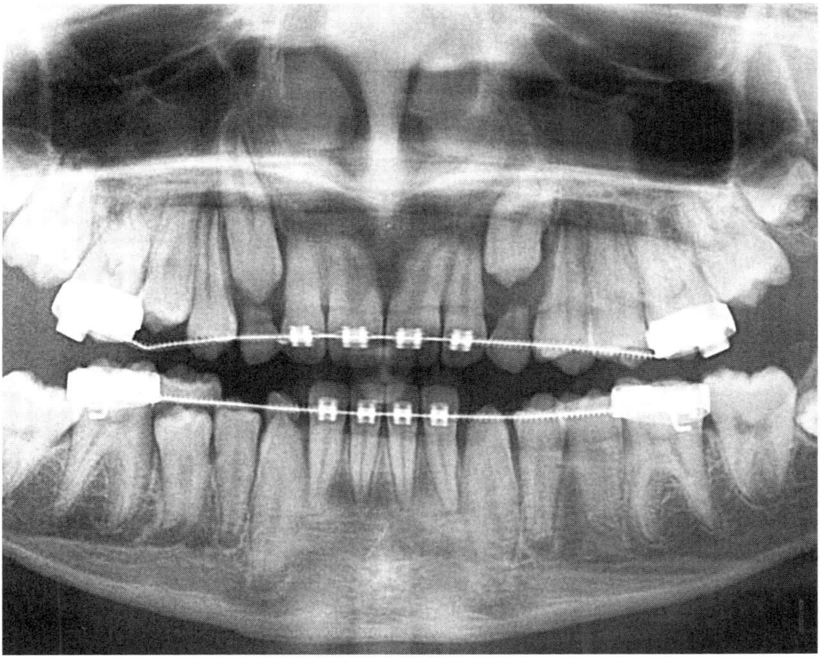

CASE STUDY 3

Justin, age 8

SITUATION

Justin's case was relatively simple. One of his upper front teeth and grown in behind the lower front teeth, and this situation had made it difficult for him to chew his food and could have resulted in damage to this tooth and surrounding gums if left alone. Justin's treatment took only six months with a few braces.

OUTCOME

Once treatment was completed, Justin had a normal

bite and did not need any further interceptive treatment. He continues to visit our office every nine months as the remainder of his permanent teeth grow in.

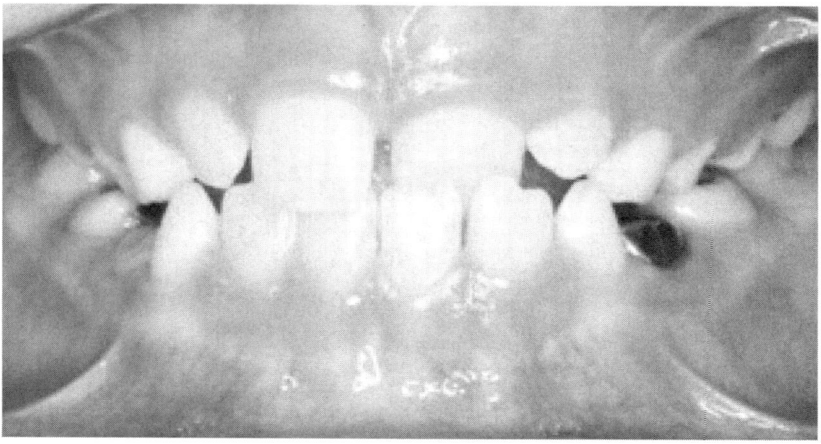

After 6 months

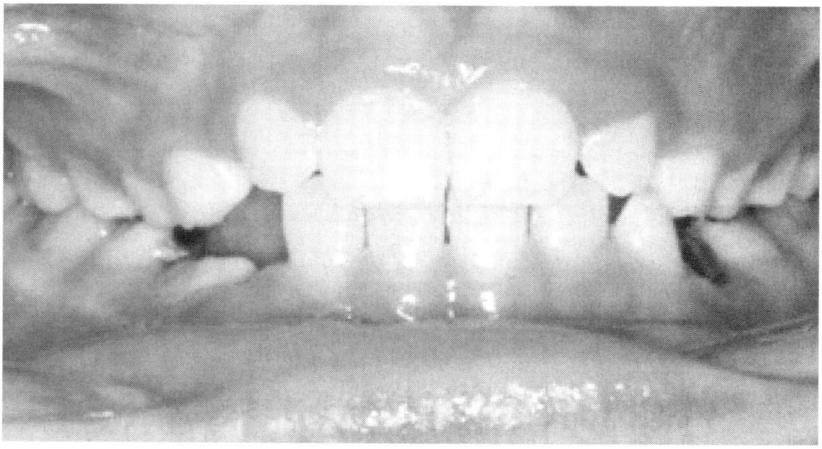

CASE STUDY 4
Brian, age 9

SITUATION

Brian had an underbite and crowding of his upper front teeth. Because his upper front teeth were behind his lower teeth, he did not have enough space for them. His treatment involved the use of braces, and expander, and rubber bands to help fix his bite.

Before

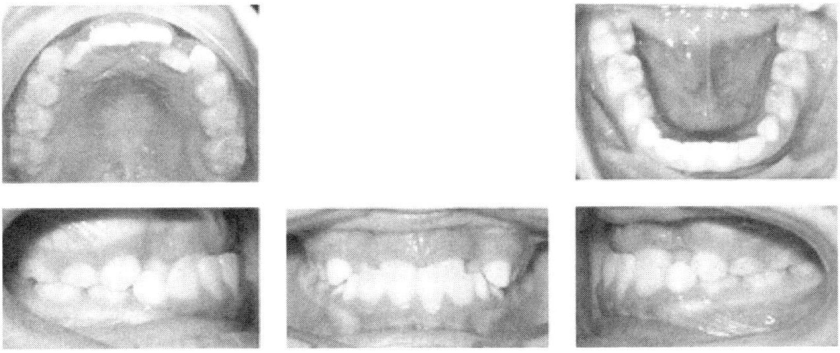

7 months

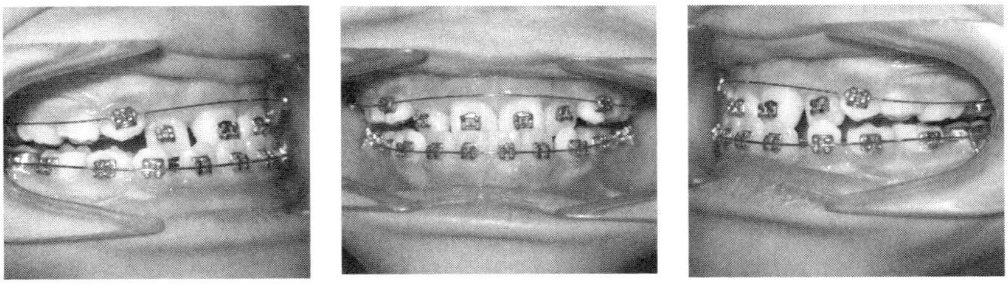

15 months

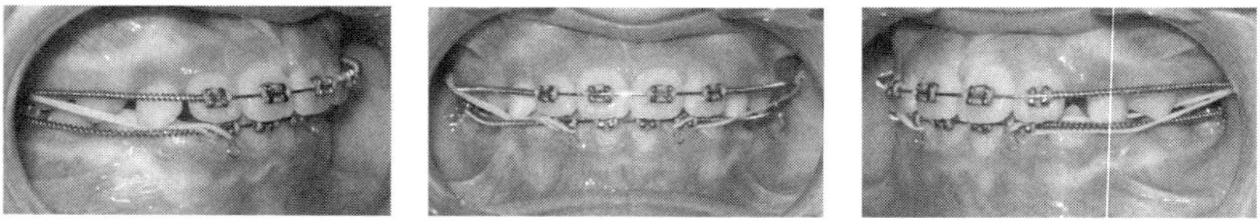

24 months

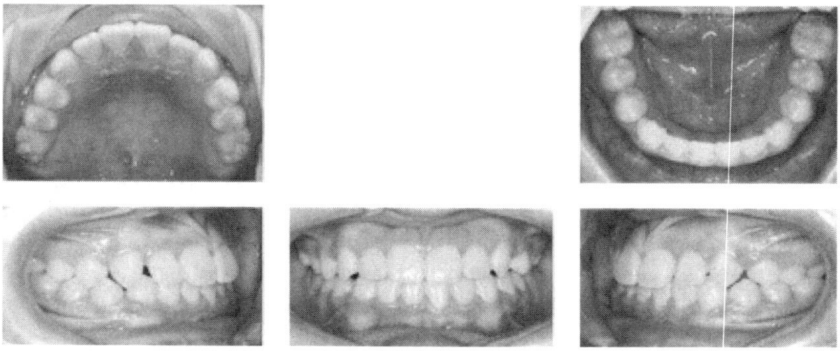

OUTCOME

10 months after the braces were removed, his teeth have almost finished growing in.

There are still a few spaces left in his upper arch that are closing as the permanent teeth continue to grow in to their final position.

CHAPTER 5
MY ORTHODONTIST TOLD ME I NEED JAW SURGERY
DR. DONNA GALANTE

"Keep smiling because life is a beautiful thing and there is so much to smile about."
Marilyn Monroe

Unless your neighbor is a surgeon who likes coming over to your house for crumpets and tea while he tells you stories about his job, you (and most people) have probably never heard the term *Orthognathic Surgery*. In this chapter, you will get to learn about all the wonders of Orthognathic Surgery, which is basically a fancy word for "Jaw Surgery".

You are probably wondering what jaw surgery entails and why it would be needed in the first place. When jaw surgery is performed, it is done to correct jaw problems that are caused by underlying skeletal deformities. Patients who usually need jaw surgery unfortunately have a bite problem that is so severe that braces alone will not suffice to correct the severe bite.

Orthognathic surgery moves your teeth and jaws into positions that are more balanced, functional and healthy. Although the goal of orthognathic surgery is to improve your bite and function, many patients also experience enhancements to their appearance, breathing and speech. The results of orthognathic surgery can have a dramatic and positive effect on many aspects of your life, and it's likely that your self-esteem and confidence will be significantly boosted.

WHY JAW SURGERY?

Jaw surgery is recommended for patients whose jaws have stopped growing. For some people, the upper jaw and lower jaw grow at different rates and the end result can be an improper or difficult bite and misaligned jaws. This makes it difficult for some people to bite and chew their food, swallow, speak or even purse their lips together. Since jaw surgery is performed to straighten jaws and orthodontics is the key to straightening teeth, the two usually go hand in hand. Parents of teenagers can rest assured though – most adolescents can avoid jaw surgery through various growth modification techniques (in conjunction with braces) or through early orthodontic intervention.

However, even with early orthodontic intervention, the jaws may still grow in a way that warrants surgery later. Many of the bite problems that require jaw surgery are genetic in origin. So if you have a family history of protruding lower jaws, there is a good chance you will have the same type of jaw structure. Early examination by an orthodontist will often provide parents and patients with an overview of how their child is growing and what the potential is for future orthodontic or jaw surgery needs will be.

An improper bite may cause various functional problems, some of which you may be experiencing right now. These problems may include chronic jaw pain (TMJ dysfunction), difficulty chewing or biting food, speech problems, unbalanced facial appearance and excessive wearing of teeth.

If you are concerned about esthetics, your orthodontist will be able to discuss your options with you and determine if braces alone will give you the look that you want, or if a combination of braces and jaw surgery is necessary.

Many patients who are candidates for jaw surgery will have recessive chins, protruding chins, gummy smiles, a smile that is off center, uneven smiles , narrow arches, protrusive upper jaws or retrusive upper jaws. All these problems can be corrected with jaw surgery and provide a huge change in not only how your bite functions, but your overall appearance.

When you go to your orthodontic consult, a thorough evaluation will be performed, which includes diagnostic records such as photos, X-rays and study models. Your orthodontist will study these records carefully and come up with a treatment plan that is personalized for you.

It is during the initial record taking and work-up that your orthodontist will determine if you need jaw surgery to get an ideal result. While surgery may be the best option to achieve the ideal result, it is an elective procedure and a treatment option that you do not have to choose. Often, there will be other treatment options presented that require no surgery but may involve a compromise in your outcome either from a cosmetic or a dental standpoint.

If jaw surgery must be performed on young children or preadolescents, it is usually done to correct congenital deformities such as cleft lip and palate. For children who are growing and have severe growth deficiencies in either the upper or lower jaw, there are several strategies that can be utilized to help aid in the growth of the affected jaw. These strategies involve wearing different devices that are generally hooked to the braces and need to be worn by the patient for long periods of time to be effective.

Cooperation is the key to success in these cases, and if cooperation is less than ideal, often the patient will not get the growth needed and will require jaw surgery later to fully correct the bite problem. Most jaw surgery is performed after the teenage growth spurt has ended. So typically for girls this would be around age 16 and for boys around ages 18 to 20.

THREE TYPES OF JAW SURGERY PROCEDURES

There are three basic types of surgical procedures. The first type of surgery is to help a patient with either a recessive chin or a protrusive chin. This operation is performed on the lower jaw (mandible) and it allows the jaw to be moved forward, thus eliminating the recessive chin. In some cases the jaw can be too far forward and this type of surgery is used to move the jaw back, which eliminates a protruding chin. The surgery is performed with no outside incisions and the mandible is rigidly fixated together so there is no need to have your teeth wired together during the healing phase.

The second procedure is performed on the upper jaw and is used for many different types of bite and cosmetic problems. It is used in situations where the patient shows a lot of upper gum tissue when they smile. It is also used when a patient has an anterior open bite (meaning their front teeth do not touch when they close down). It can also be used when a patient has an under bite (lower teeth in front of upper teeth) and the upper jaw is moved forward in this case, rather than the lower jaw being moved back.

Also, upper jaw surgery is performed to solve problems with the upper jaw being too narrow, and it is also performed on patients who have the appearance of a "short" face. The upper jaw is tilted backwards slightly to give the patient a slightly longer face.

The last procedure is called a *Genioplasty* and this operation is focused on the chin only. This procedure allows the surgeon to move a patient's chin up, forward, back, shorten it, move it down and lengthen the chin too. The choice is dependent on how you want your face and chin to look after the surgery. This is a very simple type of surgery and easiest of the three to recover from.

You might wonder what type of doctor specializes in this type of surgery. To have this surgery performed, you must be seen by an *Oral-Maxillofacial Surgeon*, and often your orthodontist will refer you to a colleague who they work closely with. It is imperative that your surgeon has an extensive background in this type of surgery.

As far as insurance coverage, this type of surgery falls under your medical plan and the surgery is performed in a hospital setting. Your surgeon and his team will be able to determine what benefits your particular medical plan has.

This is a team effort, and it is important that the patient, orthodontist and surgeon work closely together to ensure a fantastic result. Make sure you ask your surgeon about his or her experience in this type of surgery and make sure your orthodontist has a history of working on these types of cases. Sometimes a plastic surgeon may need to get involved, depending on the need for other cosmetic procedures in conjunction with the jaw surgery.

PLANNING FOR YOUR JAW SURGERY

If you are going to have jaw surgery soon or if you are contemplating having it done, here's an overview to give you a general idea of what jaw surgery involves. Generally, you will be given what is known as *Presurgerical Orthodontics* (braces or Invisalign® on your teeth) for approximately six to 18 months, depending on your treatment plan. The purpose of this phase is to align your teeth properly, so as to prepare them for surgery. Your orthodontist will know how to position your teeth to ensure that your teeth will coordinate together in an ideal way, post surgery.

Prior to surgery, your orthodontist will take updated X-rays, photos and study models, which will then be forwarded to your surgeon for an evaluation. This information will help your surgeon create a final treatment plan. Before surgery can take place, your surgeon will also need you to have a blood test, along with other types of medical tests. When you arrive at the hospital on surgery day, you will be instructed to slip into the most lovely, elegant, fashionable piece of clothing ever designed – a hospital gown – and before you know it, you will be sound asleep (thanks to the anesthesia that they give you). And once your surgery is over, you will wake up in the hospital's recovery unit.

You will have to stay at least one night in the hospital, and your surgeon will give you postoperative instructions on how to reduce the amount of swelling that occurs. Swelling can last up to six months, but it is only noticeable for approximately six weeks. Most patients will experience some pain, although it is often described as a mild soreness. Typically, it will not last more than two to three weeks, and you will be given prescription medicine to help with this soreness.

The good news about jaw surgery (other than having a newly improved jaw) is that there are no scars! All the incisions are done inside your mouth and so you do not have to worry about having scars outside or around your mouth. The biggest problem, initially, will be eating. Although your teeth will not be wired together, your jaw will be tight and you will have a new bite, which will feel different when you chew. Your doctor will give you guidelines on food that you will be allowed to eat the first few weeks after your surgery. Generally, you will stick to a soft diet and learn to love those smoothies! Since your jaw will be in the healing process, excessive chewing of hard and sticky foods will be a no-no until your surgeon directs you differently.

Most patients feel comfortable enough and are able to go back to work after a two-week recovery period. Although you may still have some swelling and won't be able to eat everything you want right away, you will soon be able to resume normal activities, with the exception of high-impact exercises. Your appearance will change a little due to the swelling, but rest assured that it is a normal part of the healing process and it will subside as you heal. If your friends and family act a little surprised at your temporary swollen look, just simply bat your eyes, tell them that they shouldn't be so jealous that they don't look as good as you and then kindly request that they fetch you lunch and give you a foot rub.

For several weeks you will not see your orthodontist and be under the surgeon's care. Once the surgeon feels that things are stable, he will refer you back to your orthodontist for the finishing phase of your orthodontic treatment.

And of course the question lingers in your mind: *"When will I get my braces off?"* Most patients will need to complete approximately three to six months of post-surgery orthodontics, during which the final positioning of the teeth is accomplished. This comprehensive approach to orthodontics involves more than just pretty teeth. It entails painstaking accuracy so as to gain the ultimate result for the patient.

The following is a testimonial from a young woman who experienced jaw surgery and wanted to share her story with you:

"Now I Can Eat Hamburgers!"

"As far as my memory reaches back, my problems with my teeth were like an invisible splinter in my finger – consistently troublesome whether I was conscious of it or not. Riding in the backseat of my mother's car on the way to school, I was drilled

over and over again on saying my S's. I didn't understand why I couldn't say them the way she wanted me to. I walked into the school's crowded hallway teary-eyed, wondering if my other classmates knew how to say their S's.

"It wasn't until I was out of elementary school that I started to really grasp what was happening. My lower jaw had grown more than it should have and the resulting under bite gave me speech difficulties. I knew I had a lisp, and when that fact was deep in my subconscious, my friends and classmates never failed to remind me of it. 'It's cute,' they would tell me, or a favorite was, 'Say stickers.' Since I had grown up with it, honestly, the lisp wasn't a problem for me.

"That is, it wasn't a problem until I wanted to be taken professionally in the work field. It shouldn't have been a problem, but I got anxious before my job interviews afraid that my lisp would be a handicap. Whether it actually affected anything, I will never know, but the uncertainty inside grew with the fact that I had a lisp. Outside the realm of work and school, the third category of my teenage life was eating. I loved to eat. I just didn't like to eat in front of other people. Since I had an under bite, my teeth weren't aligned correctly and so I had difficultly biting off pieces of food, namely sandwiches and thin noodles. I was hesitant to join my friends out to eat, especially to burger places, knowing that they would laugh at the big mess I would make while I have a whole slice of tomato hanging from my mouth.

"And pictures? Not too close please. I was always self-conscious about how my smile looked in pictures. I didn't want people to really look at me from the side either, because I was sure they would notice my jutted lower jaw. It sounds like I wouldn't have smiled at all, but the odd thing is I loved to smile and laugh, just not too close to people if they were looking. I felt like my smile was always 99-percent confident, until the miraculous day I had jaw surgery and my orthodontic work completed.

"I can't be cheesy enough when I thank my mom for taking me to the orthodontist. Now, every morning I walk through the door confident about my smile and more than willing to share it with everyone. There's an old saying that goes a smile is contagious, and I see it catching when I give a smile to the patients of the orthodontic office I work for today. And now I can eat hamburgers. No problem." – Linda S. (Age 20)

If you are in the midst of post-surgery orthodontic treatment, first of all, congratulations on coming this far! And hang in there! Your braces will soon be off; you will have a new smile, a better functioning bite and improved facial esthetics too! Jaw surgery has transformed the lives of many people and can certainly transform your smile, health and your success.

CHAPTER 6
THE FACTS, SIGNS AND SYMPTOMS OF TMJ DISORDER
DR. DONNA GALANTE

"A smile is a curve that sets everything straight."
Phyllis Diller

Perhaps you know someone who has suffered from jaw pain and tenderness located often right in front of his or her ears. You might have even experienced this type of pain yourself and had no idea, at the time, what caused this pain. The soreness and pain is located in the Temporomandibular Joint (TMJ) and the ailment associated with this joint is referred to as Temporomandibular Joint Disorder (TMJD). You're probably thinking, *"My goodness – that word is a mouthful!"*

The disorder can be more than just a mouthful, however (no pun intended). It can also be the source of unbearable pain and significant impairment to the jaw. To understand the TMJ a little better, let's first identify its location. The actual joint is essentially where your lower jaw and skull connect. This joint is what allows you to open and close your mouth, chew your food, talk, sing and yawn.

Surprisingly, however, pain and tenderness in the TMJ is quite common. The prevalence of temporomandibular joint and muscle disorder (TMJD) is between five and 12 percent. Unusual for chronic pain conditions, the prevalence rates of TMJ disorders are higher among younger persons and are at least twice as prevalent in women as men. It is estimated that for every 100 million workers in the United States, 17.8 million workdays are lost annually due to TMJ disorders, dysfunction and pain.

WHAT CAUSES TMJD?

There are many factors that could be a cause of jaw-joint pain and the associated muscle pains such as headaches and even pain in the neck and upper back areas.

Here is a list of possible causes:

- Grinding or clenching your teeth
- Arthritis in your jaw joint
- Stress
- Obstructive Sleep Apnea
- Injury to your head, neck or face from a heavy blow or whiplash injury
- Movement of the soft cushion or disc between the ball and socket of the joint due to excessive strain
- Use of oral contraceptives

WHAT ARE THE SYMPTOMS?

Common Symptoms include:

- Pain and tenderness of the jaw (typically around the ear). This pain may also radiate down the angle of the jaw.
- Ringing in the ears
- Facial pain, concentrated mostly at your jaw muscles
- Frequent headaches that vary in severity
- A bite that feels unusual – a bite that has changed in the past few months
- Difficulty in opening the mouth to chew or talk, due to pain and/or tightness in the jaw
- A tired feeling in your face
- Swelling around the jaw area
- Occasional "locking" of the jaw when it opens – there may be difficulty closing the jaw when this occurs.
- Clicking and popping sounds as the jaw opens and closes. Although these sounds alone are not detrimental, if there is pain and/or limited jaw movement associated with these sounds, it may be an indicator of TMJD.

HOW WOULD I KNOW IF I HAVE TMJD?

Patients who suffer from any or all of the aforementioned symptoms will need a comprehensive evaluation performed by a dentist or an orthodontist. They will check your jaw joints for pain or tenderness and listen for clicks, pops or grating sounds when you move them. They will also make sure your jaw is functioning properly and opens and closes in a normal fashion.

Most often they will take X-rays and photos of your teeth and bite and possibly molds of your teeth to further study how your teeth fit together and how your bite works. There may be a need for further tests such as an MRI (magnetic resonance imaging) or a CT (computer tomography scan). The MRI will show the soft tissue disc as it functions and the CT scan will show the bony details of your joints.

If your jaw pain comes and goes and seems not to affect your daily life, then you might benefit from some of the following "home" treatments to alleviate your occasional bouts of TMJD.

HOME TREATMENTS FOR TMJD

There are some things you can do to help alleviate the pain associated with TMJD.

1. You can try over-the-counter medications like naproxen or ibuprofen that can help minimize the pain and some swelling.
2. Apply an ice pack to the side of the face that is experiencing the pain and swelling for about 10 minutes. Then remove the ice pack and replace with a hot towel or washcloth to the side of your face for about FIVE minutes. Do this several times a day to help alleviate your symptoms.
3. It is always recommended to eat soft foods during an episode of jaw or facial pain. Make sure to cut your food into small pieces and chew slowly and carefully. You should avoid hard crunchy foods and eating anything that requires you to open wide. Gum chewing should be immediately discontinued at the first sign of jaw pain. This

Appointment Card
Dr. Michael Lanzetta, DDS PC 20392 Eureka Road Taylor, MI 48180 734.284.4300
Next appointment for Gavin Rose: Wed, Aug 28, 2019, 11:00 AM
If you are unable to keep an appointment, please contact our office at least 24 hours in advance.

is one habit that will increase your likelihood of further problems with your jaw joints and even more pain.

4. Definitely avoid extreme jaw movements like yawning or yelling, even singing can aggravate the situation. Also make sure to practice good posture to reduce neck and facial pain.
5. Keep your teeth slightly apart as often as you can. This will reduce the pressure on your jaw. IF you catch yourself clenching during the day, remind yourself to keep your teeth slightly apart. Sometimes holding your tongue in-between your teeth will also help in this process.
6. Finally relaxation techniques will help loosen up your jaw. Massage of the head and neck area can bring relief to your jaw and pain.

However, for many people, they suffer day in and day out not only jaw pain, but real dysfunction including the inability to chew food properly, constant facial pain, loss of sleep, excessive wear on their teeth (due to grinding), missed days of work or school, poor relationships and overall poor health.

Many TMJ problems are related to a "bad bite," and while a patient can gain temporary pain relief through use of over-the-counter medicine or some-of-the-above strategies, a consultation with a dentist or orthodontist is the best way to get to the bottom of your problem and realize a more permanent solution.

Let's praise the TM joint a little, shall we? It truly is the most unique and complex set of joints in your body. You see, each TM joint is comprised of two joints, which allow it to perform a combined rotating "hinge" action with a forward-sliding motion. The lower jaw is mostly rounded and covered with cartilage that allows your lower jaw to interact with your skull. In-between the cartilage and skull is a very thin disc that keeps the jaw moving forward as necessary. In the medical world (especially the dental world), this simple fact is one of many testaments that the human body (your body!) is remarkably built. Most people, however, are just glad that they can eat their favorite savory foods without the pains of TMJD! And that's the way it should be!

If you have suffered or are suffering from TMD, you probably want to know what treatments are available for TMD problems. The type of treatment prescribed is often dependent on the doctor's diagnosis. Once you have had a thorough evaluation by an orthodontist or dentist they will propose a treatment plan for you. Depending on the severity of your situation there are many options. Here are some of the possible treatment options. Many of these are used all together in some case for the best results.

1. **Medications.** You may need a muscle relaxer or even anti-anxiety medication to relieve stress. Higher doses of nonsteroidal anti-inflammatory drugs (NSAIDS) may be needed.
2. **Splint or Night Guard.** These are plastic mouthpieces custom-made to fit over your upper and lower teeth so they do not touch each other. This will lessen the effect of clenching or grinding. The night guards are worn only at night. However, your doctor may recommend a daytime appliance too and often these are called splints. They are

typically clear and easy-to-wear to allow for maximum compliance.

3. **Dental Work.** If you have missing teeth, crowns or bridges that are defective you may need to have these replaced in order to balance your bite.
4. **Orthodontic Treatment.** Many TMJD problems are bite-related. Deep overbites, crossbites and under bites can all cause jaw joint pain and dysfunction. Getting your bite corrected will often alleviate the pain and solve the problem permanently for you.
5. **Trigger Point Injections.** Botox or anesthesia is injected into tender facial muscles to relax the muscles and provide relief. These injections will provide temporary relief and you will need frequent injections to continue to alleviate your discomfort.
6. **Transcutaneous electrical nerve stimulation (TENS).** This therapy uses low-level electrical currents to provide pain relief by relaxing your jaw joint and facial muscles.

Even with all-the-above treatments, there are still a few patients who do not get relief from their pain and dysfunction. Often these patients will need a consultation with an oral surgeon. Further tests may need to be done in order to fully present a comprehensive plan.

The surgeon may recommend one of the following:

1. **Arthrocentesis.** This is a minor procedure that is often done in the office. Essentially you will have your jaw joint "washed" out and damaged tissue removed that may be causing some of your pain and problems.

2. **Arthroscopy.** This procedure is more invasive and requires an incision in front of your jaw joint and a special tool will be inserted so the doctor can see inside your jaw joint. This way he can determine what damage (if any) there is to the jaw joint and remove inflamed tissue or realign the disc or joint. This type of surgery leaves minimal scars and has a very short recovery time.
3. **Orthognathic surgery.** This is also known as "jaw surgery" and is often performed in conjunction with orthodontic treatment (braces or Invisalign). Based on your orthodontist's findings and treatment plan, it is determined that your jaw problem is related to how your jaws fit together. Because of a severe bite problem, you are having TMJD dysfunction and pain. Braces alone will not correct your bite problem, so your orthodontist has decided to send you for a consult with an oral surgeon. Together both doctors will work up a final treatment plan that will involve a combination of orthodontic treatment, then jaw surgery to realign the jaws into their ideal position. Often by realigning the bite this way, the jaw joints are now in a more stable and favorable position and will function better and without the previous pain and dysfunction.

CAN TMJD BE PREVENTED?

There are definitely measures you can take to avoid potential problems with your jaw joints. One was mentioned earlier and that is avoiding gum chewing. Your jaw needs to rest between meals and if you spend a good part of your day chewing gum, your jaw joints do not get the rest they need and deserve. At the first sign of jaw or facial pain, ditch the gum and see if you feel better within a few days.

Other things to avoid doing would include opening extremely wide or making your jaw move back and forth in order to make a "popping" sound. These types of movements put a lot of stress on the jaw joint and could potentially cause some problems down the road.

Wearing protective face guards when sparring in martial arts and in general avoiding any type of blow to the face or jaw. Even a soccer ball hitting your face can cause your jaw joint to be injured or even dislocated and immediately set you up for pain and dysfunction.

You need to realize that your jaw joints have a lot to do for you and you need to treat them with care and kindness. After all they work hard to help you get the nutrition you need, help you communicate with others, are useful when trying to sing or play a wind instrument, and they are responsible to helping you open up, smile and laugh.

A healthy, pain-free jaw is something that might be easily dismissed – primarily because most people are unaware of pain until it arises – but a healthy temporomandibular joint is an essential and important part of your overall smile, health and success.

CHAPTER 7
CLEAR ALIGNER TREATMENT
DR. BART BENSON

"Smile — sunshine is good for your teeth."
Author Unknown

After reading the introduction, you are aware of how a great smile can positively affect your life. You are ready to proceed to do something to straighten or align your teeth. Yet you just can't envision wearing braces.

Maybe you've done some research. Asked some friends. You've reviewed alternatives. You might be mostly concerned about your appearance, so maybe you considered clear or ceramic braces or possibly even lingual (on the inside of your teeth) braces. Clear braces are hard to see or discern from a distance so the first impression isn't always that you have metal on your teeth. Lingual braces hidden behind the teeth are difficult to discern, too, and again it's not always the first thing people see when they look at you.

Yet even with these less-visible options, something

about these braces treatment choices is still unappealing. It could be that although the ceramic or clear braces are less visible, a wire still shows. You may have concerns about embarrassment. What if a piece of food or lettuce lodges itself between your teeth and braces at an important dinner party? You might be a teenager who doesn't want to wear metal braces for your senior picture. You may have heard that the braces on the inside of your teeth (lingual braces) affect your speech so you slur your words. Lingual braces are notoriously difficult to clean. Maybe your tongue rubs against the lingual braces and causes sores.

It doesn't matter what is bothering you about these options, it's keeping you undecided to the point where your teeth aren't aligned and are not being fixed. The good news is new technology called clear-aligner therapy offers an alternative to bands, brackets and wires attached to your teeth. It's not an exclusive treatment. Almost everyone can elect to have it done.

WHAT IS CLEAR-ALIGNER THERAPY?

An alternative to metal braces, which some feel are unsightly, clear-aligner braces offer patients a less obvious method to move or guide teeth into the proper position. Clear aligners are see-through, removable plastic "trays" that go around the teeth in one continuous U-shape that resembles fake teeth or dentures. Just as traditional braces are designed to do, clear aligners use gradual force to control the movement of the teeth and properly reposition them in the mouth for a precise bite. They do not use metal bands or brackets, which are the two metal parts placed on teeth designed to fasten the wires in place. Clear aligners are made of a strong, break-resistant clear plastic. Each one is fabricated and customized to fit the individual's teeth alignment and mouth.

The goal of clear-aligner therapy and the goal of wearing braces are the same: straight teeth well-placed in your face, along with a good "bite". The goals for clear-aligner therapy versus other bite-correcting techniques including traditional braces might be the same, but the clear-aligner method is very different.

With traditional braces, you can't remove them to eat, brush, floss, play football, play the trumpet, or have perfect teeth for your senior picture. With clear-aligner therapy you have the option to remove your plastic trays. So when you eat, brush, floss, etc., your plastic trays are not in your mouth. The ability to remove your trays makes the process uniquely different and even more convenient than wearing braces.

The experience of clear-aligner therapy is very different from wearing traditional braces. Patients who select this therapy do need to realize it takes discipline not to remove the trays for extended periods of time or forget to replace them once removed. You must also be organized enough to not lose your trays when taking them out to eat, misplacing them, or leaving them somewhere. You will be expected to wear your trays all of the time unless you eat or brush your teeth. Most people do well with these expectations and are able to wear their trays approximately 22 hours per day. The longer and more you wear the trays the shorter the expected duration to wear them.

DIFFERENT TYPES OF CLEAR-ALIGNER THERAPY

There are different companies that make clear aligners. There are "red, white, and blue" aligners, Simpli-5 aligners, Clear Correct aligners, MTM aligners, and more. The most famous because of the extensive advertisements is Invisalign®.

In 1945, Dr. Harold Kesling published a paper in the *Journal of Orthodontics and Oral Surgery* where he envisioned "creating some simple appliance that would influence all of the teeth to flow into their best possible position with relation to one another without any interference from bands or wires."

Dr. Kesling dreamed of creating an appliance like Invisalign, but the technology in 1945 was insufficient to make this a practical reality. In the 1990's there was a person by the name of Zia Chishti. Zia had worn braces in his early 20's and had not enjoyed the experience. After having his braces removed, he was given clear retainers to wear at night. Zia noticed if he skipped a night of wearing his retainers his teeth would begin to go crooked. He also noticed that if he wore his retainers for a few days after skipping a night or two of retainers wear, his teeth would re-align. This made him wonder if there was a way of aligning teeth without wearing braces.

As was the case with Dr. Kesling, Zia needed technology to make his vision come to reality. However, the difference between 1995 and 1945 was computer technology. You could now create digital images of someone's teeth and digitally straighten them. So with computer-aided design and computer-aided manufacturing (CAD/CAM) Invisalign was created. In 1999 Invisalign treatment was introduced as a way to straighten your teeth without wearing braces.

HOW DOES INVISALIGN WORK?

Using either a highly accurate impression of your teeth or a scanned image, digital representations are made of your teeth. Technicians use the computer to manipulate the digital representation to move your digital teeth a tiny amount. This tiny sum represents the amount of aligning one tray can accomplish.

Then a tray customized to correspond with the digital image is created and matched to the mouth. Your orthodontist confirms the tray fits as intended and explains how to wear and take care of your tray. You are asked to wear that particular tray 22 hours per day for two weeks. Then the process is repeated over and over again. The technician moves your digital teeth a tiny amount on screen. A new custom tray is made. It's put back in your mouth. You wear it. It does its job and moves the teeth – repeat until your digital teeth and real-life teeth are straight.

Each time your digital teeth are moved by a technician, this represents a stage or a single tray that when placed in your mouth will move your teeth. If the technician has to move your teeth 26 times to align your digital teeth, this represents 26 trays that you will need to wear to align your teeth. Since each tray or aligner is worn approximately 22 hours a day for two weeks, 26 trays (52 weeks) would represent a year's worth of treatment with Invisalign. The only thing you need to remember is follow your orthodontist's directions and wear your trays as instructed.

ADVANTAGES OF INVISALIGN

You will discover many wonderful advantages to using clear-aligner therapy. These advantages and benefits are specific to this technology and include:

- Attractive Esthetics
- Improved Comfort
- More Convenience
- Improved Oral Hygiene

Esthetics

The most noticeable advantage of Invisalign compared to traditional metal braces is the fact the wearing Invisalign is almost invisible. Hence the name, Invisalign, meaning you can align your teeth almost invisibly. The clear trays are hardly noticeable by the average person. Many people don't want the "glaring" and obvious wires on their teeth. Older people who don't want to feel like they're back to their teenage years especially don't want visible braces. People whose image is dependent somehow on their looks often avoid traditional braces.

There are many people today enjoying benefits of clear-aligner therapy, which includes:

- Increased self-confidence
- For single people perhaps a new romantic partner
- A promotion at work (e.g., maybe selling more real estate because of a new smile).

These people would not have considered wearing braces to improve their smiles. Wearing traditional metal braces would be too noticeable, but with the option of wearing Invisalign they chose to straighten their teeth. Unless someone is close enough to be in your personal space, the aligners or trays that you wear are not noticeable.

One of the nicest benefits esthetically speaking is for those who have spaces or gaps between their teeth. Using Invisaligners to close the spaces immediately proves beneficial to appearance. As you put your first tray in and begin to wear them the space appears smaller. This is due to the way light reflects off the plastic trays. It's like an optical illusion! There are millions of people who have straightened their teeth using Invisalign who would have never made the decision to have treatment if their only option was traditional metal braces.

Comfort

As an orthodontist Dr. Benson has adolescents and adults ask: Does it hurt to get braces placed on your teeth?

Dr. Benson answers that it is usually not painful to have braces placed on your teeth. There are no needles, drills or shots that are needed to put braces on. In the past when a band (which is like a ring around your tooth) was put on every tooth it was much more uncomfortable, but today most teeth just need brackets bonded to the surface of the tooth. This makes getting braces a much easier and more comfortable process.

In order to have braces placed or bonded on your teeth, your teeth need to be dry. Your mouth is not normally a dry environment. So to isolate your teeth from your saliva, a device is placed that prevents your lip, cheeks, tongue, and saliva from touching your teeth. We call the device a "cheek retractor". It is not sharp and does not cut or poke you, but some people find it slightly uncomfortable. But once you have adapted to the cheek retractor, having the braces placed on your teeth is not painful.

If you choose Invisalign treatment, there is no need for

a cheek retractor. You either need to have an impression (or mold) of your teeth or you need to have a digital scan made of your teeth. People who gag easily may find the impressions uncomfortable, but if your orthodontist has a digital scanner you do not have to worry about having the "goopy" impression material placed in your mouth.

The digital intraoral scanner is a new technology that has several advantages over impressions. (I discuss scanning of your teeth later in this chapter.) Advantages to the patient experience include elimination of the discomfort of impressions or re-impressions. It shortens appointment duration and reduces return appointments. It's a powder-free process, which improves patient comfort and it provides real-time visualization for the orthodontist to educate patients right on the spot.

DOES STRAIGHTENING YOUR TEETH WITH BRACES HURT?

Most people are sore for two to three days after having the braces attached to their teeth. To make teeth move, pressure has to be applied. The pressure and your body's reaction to the pressure is one of the reasons your teeth get sore.

The pressure is not the only thing you have to adapt to. All of the brackets, bands and wires are not perfectly smooth. Although a lot of effort is put into making the braces small and smooth, the brackets still have corners and angles. A certain amount of tenderness is to be expected. Your mouth may ache, and over-the-counter aspirin, Tylenol or ibuprofen reduces tenderness and pain. You may have heard of people putting wax on their brackets or braces. This makes the braces feel smoother. Some people have to use wax on their braces for days or weeks. Eventually your mouth toughens up, similar to the way your hands or feet develop calluses.

Also eating will be different with braces. Braces are great at collecting food. After you eat a meal with braces on your teeth, look in the mirror. You may see a lot of what you just ate is attached to your braces. You will need to spend more time brushing your teeth with braces and you may need special cleaning equipment such as a water pick to thoroughly rinse and clean your braces of unsightly debris left in your teeth and for dental health.

Having braces on your teeth is a lot to get used to.

With Invisalign treatment the above does not happen. The amount of force placed on your teeth by your plastic Invisalign trays is much less than the amount of force placed on your teeth by braces. The plastic trays can only apply so much force. Wires and braces can apply significantly more force to your teeth. Since the plastic Invisalign trays apply less force, your teeth do not get as sore. Your teeth will still have some slight pressure applied to them so they will move. So the first day of Invisalign treatment you may experience some soreness. Most people take ibuprofen or Tylenol (as noted for traditional braces, too) for a day or so to take the "edge" off. Some people admit they never get sore.

Every two weeks as you put in your new tray, you will notice the trays are tighter and you may experience some mild soreness, but the first tray is usually the one that people notice. Another way to think about this is when you get braces "tightened" or adjusted, your orthodontist applies enough force for a four-week or possibly even an eight-week interval. But with Invisalign you do your own tightening every two weeks when you put the new tray or aligner in and the plastic Invisalign trays are only designed to apply enough force for a two-week interval. This translates into a lower force than metal braces and therefore less discomfort.

Another difference in the comfort levels is the way Invisaligners feel as compared to traditional metal braces. Braces have corners and edges, but Invisalign trays are smooth. As you run your tongue around the plastic trays, you will not notice the roughness that you feel with braces. You will not need to use wax. Occasionally there may be an edge of the plastic that rubs your lip. If that occurs I recommend people use a fingernail file to smooth the rough edge. Overall it is much easier to get used to the feel of Invisaligners compared to traditional metal braces.

When it comes to eating with Invisalign treatment, you remove the trays to eat. So there is no food that gets stuck or trapped in your braces, and there are no dietary restrictions as there are with braces. You can eat whatever you desire and not worry about breaking anything or having food stuck to your braces.

Convenience

We live in a fast-paced world. Whether you are a teenager who can't miss school, plays after-school sports, or has other after-school activities, or an adult who does not want to take time off from work, everyone is busy. If there were a way to put braces on your teeth and come back in 18 months to have the braces removed, orthodontists would be doing this. Unfortunately this is not how braces work.

Braces require adjusting or tightening to align your teeth. This means monthly or bi-monthly visits to see your orthodontist. You could also have unplanned or emergency visits due to a wire poking you, a bracket that may have come loose, or other unanticipated problems. When you choose Invisaligners as your treatment you will have fewer visits. There are no wires to poke your cheeks or lips. There are no brackets to come loose. In fact most of my Invisalign patients finish their treatment faster than my braces patients.

Invisalign treatment also fits your lifestyle. If you have to speak in public, you may be self-conscious speaking with braces, but with Invisalign treatment if you were nervous about speaking with the plastic trays in (even though they are almost invisible) you can remove them. If you are getting married and don't want anything on your teeth for your wedding photographs you can take your Invisalign trays out for the photographs. Your job may require you to travel and you may be away from home for months at a time, then your orthodontist can give you enough trays to last until you are back home.

The same scenario applies to college students who attend school hundreds of miles away from home. If they had braces on their teeth and had a bracket come loose, they may not be able to come back home to have their orthodontist resolve the issue. They may not be able to make their normal adjustment visits thereby slowing down their treatment progress. But with Invisalign treatment your orthodontist can give you enough plastic trays to last for your semester. You won't have to worry about something breaking or poking you while you are away at school.

Perhaps you are in high school and don't want your senior picture to show you with braces on your teeth. Maybe you play a wind instrument in the band or play sports and are worried about getting your lips smashed against the metal braces. You can remove Invisalign and avoid those potential hazards.

For all of these reasons and more, choosing to straighten your teeth using Invisaligners is the most convenient method available.

Oral Hygiene

Oral hygiene is the term dental professionals use when discussing keeping your teeth clean. It involves brushing and flossing your teeth to remove all of the food after eating. With conventional metal braces, it is a challenge to keep your teeth clean and free of food and dental plaque (plaque is a sticky substance that builds up on your teeth after eating). The braces tend to accumulate food around them and underneath the wire. It takes extra effort to remove all of the food and plaque from around your braces. It can be done but does take more time and effort with braces on.

Unfortunately, there a lot of children, adolescents and even some adults who struggle with doing an adequate job keeping their braces and teeth clean of food and plaque. When your teeth and braces have plaque and food attached to them your body experiences inflammation. Your gums will get red, swollen, and may even bleed. This is called gingivitis. Gingivitis is a reversible condition. Once the braces are removed and you are able to brush and floss your teeth adequately, the inflammation will subside. This may take a couple of months, but the normal pink color will return, the swelling will shrink, and your gums will no longer bleed.

There is something else that occurs to people wearing braces who have poor oral hygiene. When dental plaque stays on your teeth, naturally occurring oral bacteria use the dental plaque as a food source. After ingesting the dental plaque the bacteria excrete what they don't eat on your teeth. This bacterial excretion is an acid, and if the acid stays on your teeth long enough the enamel of your tooth becomes decalcified. Decalcified enamel is very white. It is as white as the paper this book is written on. Your teeth are not this white. You may have seen someone who has worn braces and has these "white spots" (areas of enamel decalcification) on their teeth. Usually the decalcified areas are around the periphery of where the bracket was on the tooth. The most common areas for enamel decalcification to occur are on your upper front teeth – the teeth that are most visible when you smile. Unlike gingivitis, which is a reversible condition, enamel decalcification is not reversible. Your teeth will be permanently scarred if this occurs.

The great news is with Invisalign treatment, this very rarely occurs because there are no braces to collect food and no braces to brush around. You continue to brush and floss as you normally would. This makes it much easier to have good oral hygiene and avoid gingivitis and enamel decalcification.

CAN MY TEETH BE STRAIGHTENED USING INVISALIGN?

When Invisalign first came out, it was a new technology. Like many new technologies there were some issues or "bugs" to work out. Although it was the most sophisticated method available, it was still a young and relatively unproven technology. In the early years of Invisalign's existence, it was designed for adults only. It was also designed for relatively easy cases. If you had worn braces as an adolescent, but had neglected to wear your retainers as instructed, your teeth may have crowded again. Orthodontists call this "relapse" meaning your teeth had moved back to where they originally were before braces. If your teeth had not relapsed too far, you were a good candidate for Invisalign treatment.

Slightly spaced or slightly crooked teeth with relatively good "bites" were the type of cases that the early rendition of Invisalign was designed to treat. As orthodontists and the Invisalign Company (Align Technology) gained more experience, it became apparent that the plastic trays had difficulty straightening some teeth. If your teeth were turned or rotated and the shape of the tooth was very round, then aligning the rotated tooth using Invisaligners was not very successful.

Occasionally patients would have to have metal braces put on their teeth to achieve straight teeth. No one was satisfied with this situation, so research into how to move teeth with plastic trays was started. The research found that some of the movements required an "attachment" to be placed on the tooth. An attachment is a tooth-colored "bump" of composite material that is bonded to your tooth. One of the reasons that an attachment may be needed is that the plastic tray has no flat surface on the tooth to "push" against. In the example of a very round tooth that needs rotational correction, the plastic would push against the curved surface of the tooth. Instead of the tooth moving, the plastic would just slip off the tooth. So research was done on how to modify the tooth's surface so the plastic tray has something to push against.

The method Align Technology devised was to bond some tooth-colored composite material on the tooth so when the plastic tray applied force to rotate the tooth it would have a surface to apply force to. Then instead of the plastic tray slipping off the tooth, the tooth would move. Sometimes a tooth might be tilted, meaning it leans to the left or the right. Or if it is a back tooth it may lean forward or backward. Correcting a tooth that is tilted may also require attachments. Sometimes correcting a tilted tooth requires two attachments. If you need two attachments on a tooth to correct a tilt issue, don't worry – the attachments are small.

You might be surprised by the amount of time, energy and effort that goes into designing the attachments' shape. Align technology has hired some of the preeminent experts in the field of orthodontic biomechanics. These experts know the amount and direction of force needed to move teeth in a certain direction. They have researched what the size and shape of attachments should be in order to apply the correct amount and direction of force to an individual tooth.

As an example every canine tooth has a similar shape, but they are individual teeth each with its own distinctive size and shape. The attachment shape that may work on a small canine tooth may be too small to rotate a large canine tooth that has an unusual shape. So each attachment is designed to fit a particular tooth according to its size and shape and by which direction it needs to move.

Invisalign therapy is very individualized. The attachments are designed for the size and shape of your teeth. Your trays only fit your teeth. They are not like a pair of shoes where you know you wear a certain size and that size shoe is mass-produced at a factory in Asia. Your treatment is designed for your particular condition and your specific teeth. Invisalign is a miracle of mass production of individualized, custom-designed products. It would be like you were measured or had your body scanned for every pair of shoes or article of clothing that you wore. This is what Invisalign is like.

Occasionally a patient says that an attachment on a front tooth is visible. It's understandable that the patient doesn't like it and wishes the attachment was not needed. But if they want their front tooth to become straight then an attachment may be required. Patients should know that the attachment is much less noticeable than the smallest bracket or brace. So if you want your teeth to align, you may need some attachments bonded to your teeth.

The researchers at Align Technology know that attachments are not popular, so they are investigating ways that a tooth can be moved without attachments. One of the ways that they have discovered is that instead of changing the shape of the tooth by bonding an attachment to it, they can alter the shape of the plastic. For example, this works if your front teeth lean inward. In these cases an indentation is built into the plastic. This indentation is called a "power ridge". The power ridge applies pressure to the part of the tooth closest to your gums. By applying pressure in this location, researchers have determined that the correct amount and direction of force can be created to change the inward-leaning front tooth. It is hoped as further research occurs into the forces created by these indentations of plastic that more of these power ridges instead of attachments can be used to move teeth in the desired direction.

Another innovation that is now available with Invisalign treatment is the ability to treat overbites and underbites. In the early years of Invisalign's existence, correcting overbites (more accurately called "overjet" by orthodontists), which occurs when the upper front teeth stick out in front of the bottom front teeth, or underbites (lower front teeth stick out in front of upper front teeth) was not possible. If you wanted your overbite or underbite corrected you had to wear braces.

If you were wearing braces in order to correct your bite problem, there is a good chance your orthodontist would ask you to wear elastics or rubber bands that would stretch from your bottom braces to your top braces. You can now do the same thing with Invisalign. You attach the rubber bands to a notch cut into the plastic or to a small brace bonded to the tooth.

Patients are usually surprised by this possibility. Having this innovation available increases the number and type of cases that can be treated using Invisalign. Before this innovation was available your orthodontist may have informed you that your teeth or your bite could not be corrected with Invisalign. But if you follow your orthodontist's directions regarding how and for how long to wear the elastics (rubber bands) you can achieve a correction of your overbite or underbite. Of course not all overbites or underbites are the same. If you have a severe bite problem, braces and possibly even jaw surgery may be needed.

CAN TEENAGERS USE INVISALIGN TO STRAIGHTEN TEETH?

When Invisalign was first introduced it was only for adults. Adults make up about 20-25 percent of people who are undergoing orthodontic treatment. This leaves 75 to 80 percent of people undergoing orthodontic treatment out of luck if they wanted to use Invisalign as the method to align their teeth.

This left a lot of teens who wanted to use Invisalign instead of braces to align their teeth disappointed. They wanted to use Invisalign instead of braces for the same reasons as adults. They did not want people to notice they were wearing braces. They were concerned about wearing braces and playing sports. What would happen if they were hit in their mouthes playing their favorite sports? They did not want to have their mouth cut up when their lips got smashed against the braces. Perhaps they had a speaking part in the school play or played a wind instrument like the trumpet in the school band. Would they still be able to press the mouthpiece of the trumpet against their lips and braces and play? If they were playing the part of an adult in the school play, what would it look like if they were wearing braces?

What about the senior picture? Taking a senior picture is a big milestone in a teen's life. Parents ask all of the time if the braces will be off in time for the senior pictures. If you are an adult, you may have forgotten what your senior picture looked like, but for many teens at that point in their lives the senior picture is a major milestone. It is the picture that parents put in the den or family room. It is the picture you see when you go back for your class reunion. It is the picture that follows you for your entire life.

So there was a desire from teens to wear Invisalign, but if you were the parent of a teen, you may have some questions like: Will my teen be responsible enough to wear the trays as instructed? Will my teen lose the trays? Teenagers are not all alike. Some are very responsible and some are not. Some follow directions and some do not. When parents ask if Invisalign is the right choice for their child the answer is that some of the best Invisalign patients are teenagers. If they have a child who wants their teeth straight but the teen does not want to wear braces, then their child will do great with Invisalign because they are motivated.

When Align Technology decided to make Invisaligners for teens they modified the product in order to address parental concerns. The product is called Invisalign Teen. There are some innovations that make the Invisalign Teen product different than Invisalign for adults. The items that make the teen product different are:

Wear Indicators. The wear indicators are blue dots built into each of the Invisalign plastic trays. When you take the Invisalign tray out of the packaging the wear-indicator dot is dark blue. As the Invisalign tray is worn 22 hours per day for two weeks, the dark-blue dot becomes a faded-blue dot. The wear indicator is there so parents can monitor their child wearing his/her aligners Mom or Dad can look at a tray that has been worn for two weeks and compare it to the next new tray to be worn. Then they can tell if it has been worn by comparing the color of the wear-indicator dots of the old Invisalign tray to the wear-indicator dot of the new Invisalign tray.

Free replacement aligners. When I am consulting with parents regarding their child wearing Invisaligners, one of the comments I often hear is "Susie can't keep up with her glasses, contacts, books, homework, etc." With Invisalign Teen, their child can lose up to six sets of Invisalign trays and receive six upper and lower replacement trays at no additional charge.

Altering of adjusting treatment for baby teeth that may still be present is another feature of the Invisalign Teen product. Some children slowly lose their baby teeth. If your teen is like this, he or she can still wear Invisaligners. Invisalign Teen makes allowances for the loss of the baby teeth and the eruption of the permanent tooth that will take the place of the baby tooth.

THE INTRA-ORAL SCANNER

In order to manufacture plastic trays that fit your teeth, Align Technology has to have an accurate image of your teeth. One of the ways of obtaining an image of your teeth is to have an impression made.

Using a tray that holds impression material makes an impression. Impression materials come in different colors and viscosities and have different setting times. The setting time means: how long does the impression have to stay in your mouth to set or become semi-rigid? When an impression is made of your teeth, the impression material is initially flow-able or semi-liquid. It is thicker than water. Imagine a thick syrupy molasses. The material has to flow around your teeth to capture all of the curves, crevices and contours of your teeth and the surrounding gums. If you have had dental work like a crown or a cap of one of your teeth, then you have had an impression.

Impressions have been used a long time in dentistry to produce a replica of patient's teeth. The impression is a negative image of your teeth, gums and jawbone. This negative image is converted into a positive image by pouring a plaster-like substance into the impression, which then hardens into a replica of your teeth, gums and jawbone. If you are a fan of crime shows like CSI then you may have seen police technicians make impressions of tire tracks or footprints in order to solve a crime.

Impressions are used in a variety of ways and in different industries. Impressions are used in dentistry to make dentures, partials, crowns, veneers, bleaching trays, mouthpieces, retainers, and the list goes on. Most people do not have a problem with impressions, but if you have a very sensitive gag reflex, then having an impression made of your teeth can be an unpleasant experience. I have seen many patients vomit while an impression is being made of their mouths and teeth. No one wants to go to the orthodontist's office to vomit, and the orthodontic team does not want to cause someone to vomit or clean the mess up. It is really a yucky experience to be avoided if you can.

Thanks to modern technology, you can avoid the impression. Instead of having an impression made of your teeth and gums, you can have your teeth and gums scanned. Scanning technology has been around for decades. You may have scanned a document into your computer. Scanning involves making a digital image of something. It is like taking a picture of a letter. Well, it is now possible to scan or obtain three-dimensional digital images of your teeth.

If you are one of those people who gag easily then the intra-oral scanner is made for you. You won't have the urge to gag like you do with a tray of "goopy" impression material dripping down your throat. Not only is the digital intraoral scanner more comfortable, it is more accurate. An impression of your teeth is a "negative" image of your teeth that has to be converted into a "positive" image of your teeth. This is similar to film photography, when you had to get your film developed from a negative into your printed photographs. The transformation of the impression of your teeth into a digital image of your teeth is likely to introduce small distortions. These distortions mean that your Invisalign trays don't fit onto your teeth as well as they could.

If you have your teeth scanned instead of having an impression made of your teeth, then there is no negative image of your teeth that has to be converted into a "positive" image of your teeth. The slight distortions of your teeth that are inherent in the impression process are also not present. So what does this mean to you? It means that your Invisalign trays will fit your teeth better, and your teeth will align more efficiently if your teeth have been scanned instead of having an impression made of your teeth.

You also will receive your trays or aligners quicker if your teeth are scanned as opposed to having an impression. Your impressions have to be mailed to the company that makes your aligner trays, which is Align Technology. They are mailed using a delivery service like United Parcel Service to transport your impressions to Costa Rica. Costa Rica is the country where the technicians transform the impressions of your teeth from a "negative" image into a positive image. But if you have your teeth scanned, the digital images of your teeth and gums are sent within minutes to Align Technology. This saves time on shipping. It is a positive image of your teeth and gums. No technician has to convert a negative image into a positive image, which also saves time.

Another advantage of the digital intraoral scanner as compared to impressions is you can see a prediction of what your teeth will look like straight the day your teeth are scanned. Many people find this to be rewarding and motivating. Dr. Benson often uses words in an attempt to paint a word picture of what a prospective patient's teeth will look like straight. Many times I find my words inadequate. There is a reason for the expression, "A picture is worth a thousand words." Once they see the image of their teeth straight, people are encouraged to begin orthodontic treatment. They have a fuller understanding of the end results, much more than words can convey. They are also excited to see what they are working toward – a perfect smile.

THE FUTURE OF CLEAR-AIGNER THERAPY

Today there are still people who want to straighten their teeth with Invisalign but are not candidates. There are still conditions that require braces to correct. If you have a tooth that is in your gums that will not erupt, your teeth are so crooked that you need four teeth removed, if you have a severe bite problem, and other conditions too numerous to mention, then you may need braces to resolve your particular problem.

To some degree it involves the distance your teeth must move to become straight. Your teeth have roots that you can't see. Most of your tooth is the root. The length of the root is longer than the crown of your tooth (the crown of your tooth is what you see in your mouth). If your teeth have to move a long distance to become straight, then the roots of your teeth have to move that distance. Moving roots of teeth long distances is difficult even with braces, but it is exceptionally difficult with Invisalign treatment.

As orthodontists gain more experience treating difficult cases with Invisalign and the researchers at Align Technology continue to improve the product, then hopefully some of the conditions that Invisalign treatment cannot treat today can be treated using this product in the future.

If you see an orthodontist who tells you that Invisalign won't work for you and you need braces, ask him how many cases he has done using Invisalign. The orthodontist who has more experience with Invisalign will have more knowledge and skill treating difficult cases with Invisalign. Orthodontics is a field where different doctors have different opinions about Invisalign treatment.

YOU DESERVE A PERFECT SMILE

With all of the physical and emotional barriers gone to getting braces by using Invisalign, why not? Don't you deserve to have a beautiful, perfect smile to light up the room? If you do things like cover your mouth when you laugh, feel embarrassed over those crooked teeth, or have an overbite or underbite, don't despair any longer. You don't always have to have a mouthful of metal to correct your smile.

Now with Invisalign treatment you can avoid the unsightly problems of metal brackets and wire. You can instead have clear-plastic trays that are hardly noticeable. You can enjoy a more convenient and comfortable process. You can see well in advance what you're working toward. You can still enjoy those activities braces would get in the way of doing. And when you're finished you can smile big, wide and proud that you have the teeth you only dreamed possible!

Don't you deserve that smile? Yes, you do!

CHAPTER 8
RETAINERS AND THE IMPORTANCE OF RETENTION
DR. MICHAEL LANZETTA

"Smile, it lets your teeth breathe."
Author Unknown

In love with his profession and fortunate to work in a field that allows him to improve patients' health while helping them have more success in life through better self-esteem and greater confidence – that is what Dr. Michael Lanzetta enjoys.

Dr. Lanzetta, AKA Dr. Mike to most people, is a lifelong resident of Michigan. He was born in Detroit, and he has spent his entire life growing up and living in suburban Detroit. He has been married to his wife Elana for 33 years, and they have two daughters, Jenna, 22, and Samantha, 19. Jenna graduated from Western Michigan, and Samantha is in her second year at Michigan State. They live in Belleville. His hobbies include photography and aviation. He flies his own plane, and when possible, he rescues dogs through the Pilots-N-Paws program.

Dentistry, and especially orthodontics can be considered part science/medicine and part art. There is an artistic, creative side to orthodontics that drew Dr. Lanzetta in many years ago. He knew he wanted to be a dentist as far back as high school. He has always loved working with his hands, and science was always his favorite subject. Dr. Lanzetta graduated from the University of Michigan Dental School in 1985 and the University of Indiana Orthodontic program in 1987. He has been practicing in Taylor for over 25 years.

Dr. Lanzetta is passionate about providing excellent results and superior experiences. His overriding philosophy of orthodontics is to minimize treatment. At all times, he wants to design each patient's treatment to take as little time as possible and use fewer appliances. This may mean delaying treatment, since too often braces are placed before all adult teeth are in, which makes the patient wait an extra amount of time to finish. He also uses the most advanced braces available, which shortens the treatment time even further. He is also excited about all of the new technologies available today to help make his patients' experiences the best possible.

He is also passionate about helping you keep your teeth straight once they've been finished – and that is what this chapter is all about. The day you finish treatment and look in the mirror to see a beautiful set of teeth staring back at you is truly a wonderful moment. Maintaining those beautiful teeth is called retention. There are many common misconceptions about retention, and this chapter will attempt to sort it out for you. One thing is certain, as Dr. Lanzetta frequently explains, after straightening your teeth, your teeth absolutely will not stay straight without retention.

RETAINERS AND RETENTION

So what is retention? Retention is the use of appliances to keep teeth from undesirable movements. This could mean holding spaces open while waiting for adult teeth to erupt in, holding expansion that has occurred from an expansion appliance, holding teeth from drifting as other teeth come in, or holding teeth in their final positions.

In order to do this, orthodontics use what are called retainers. Dr. Lanzetta makes custom-fitted acrylic or wire appliances that place just enough pressure to prevent teeth from moving. Before talking about how all of this works, it is important to understand that orthodontists also use retainers to move teeth.

The word retainer is one of those words that has become so common that it can very easily be misunderstood. A retainer is specifically any appliance made out of acrylic or wires used to hold teeth. Because orthodontists are so familiar with retainers, they have learned how to modify them to actually move teeth. Using retainers as such a tool, your orthodontist also sometimes will use "retainers" to move teeth. That's right, orthodontists use a device that was meant for holding teeth to move teeth. There are two specific situations Dr. Lanzetta is going to mention in this chapter since he often uses them.

1. A small adjustable wire, called a finger spring, is added to an otherwise normal retainer. This is often used during First Phase (a time when a person still has baby teeth and

thus is not ready for full braces) to gently tip a tooth or two for a particular need. This appliance then is an active appliance, yet looks like a regular old retainer. This is where the confusion comes in as orthodontists are using something to move teeth when it is normally thought of as only being able to hold teeth. Dr. Lanzetta uses retainers for small movements in First-Phase treatment instead of braces because it is simpler, less expensive, and easier for young patients to tolerate. Once you realize that you can make modifications to a retainer, you are only limited by your imagination as to how it's used. This is the part of orthodontics that rests solidly in the art and creativity area just referred to earlier.

2. Extra acrylic is added to an upper retainer right behind the front incisors in the shape of a flat plane. Imagine a normal retainer, only one with thicker acrylic just behind the upper front teeth. This is used to open or reverse a deep bite. A deep bite exists when the lower incisors over erupt and start to occlude well up into the area close to the roof of the mouth or palate. In more severe cases, the lower incisors can sometimes even touch the palate. By placing extra acrylic behind the incisors, the lower incisors are prevented from further over eruption. What's more, because the upper and lower back teeth are not allowed to touch each other, they start to erupt toward each other. This movement has the effect of further opening the bite. Opening a very deep bite while using braces can be challenging and time-consuming. Opening the bite prior to using braces can be more effective, shortening the time necessary for braces later.

THE THREE MOST COMMON TYPES OF RETAINERS

There are three main types of retainers: Hawley, Essix, and Bonded Lingual Hawley.

Hawley

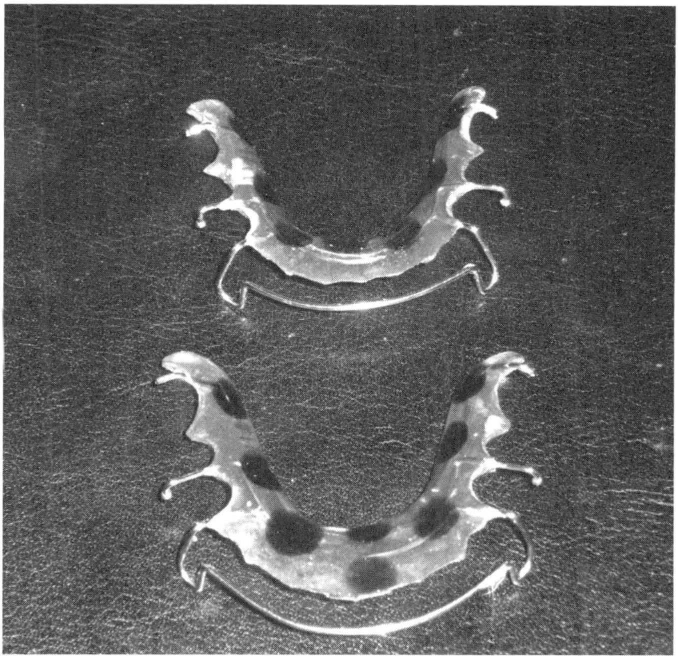

This is the most traditional type. It has been around the longest, and it is the most widely used retainer. It is made of acrylic formed to the inside surfaces of the teeth (the side the tongue touches), and has an outer wire called a Labial Bow that touches the outer surfaces (the side the lips touch). It has a wire hook or clasp to help hold it onto the teeth, and a small wire toward the back that sits near the biting surface of the molar to prevent the retainer from over-seating or getting pushed into the gums.

Why would orthodontists use a Hawley? This retainer has many advantages, including durability, repair-ability and customizability. Dr. Lanzetta can add designs and colors to it, and he can realign teeth to a limited degree.

The main advantages of this retainer are its durability and customizability. This is one tough retainer. It takes a lot to break it. As such, with proper wear and a touch of care, it can last up to 10 years. It is not indestructible, however, and over the years Dr. Lanzetta has seen his patients go to great lengths to find creative ways to kill it. One patient told the doctor his retainer got run over by a cement truck. It did not survive. Leaving it behind in a restaurant or an enthusiastic and hungry dog are the two most common ways to part company with a Hawley. Stories of families "dumpster diving" for a lost retainer are legendary.

When it does break, it can very often be repaired. In Dr. Lanzetta's office, there is no charge to repair a broken Hawley. Two important conditions must apply:

1. It first has to be reparable. One clean break of the acrylic or a broken wire is reparable. If it is broken in multiple locations and the wires are bent, chances are it is not reparable.
2. It has to fit. As this chapter will discuss, retainers will continue to fit well when they are worn properly, and for every day that goes by without wearing them, they become increasingly harder to get in. If you wait too long to come in for a repair, they simply will not fit, and so they cannot be repaired.

Over the years Dr. Lanzetta has devised many ways to modify the Hawley retainer. Besides changing the acrylic by adding colors and even small designs and logos, the plastic and the wires can be modified to institute small movements of the teeth. Tiny auxiliary wires called Finger Springs can be added to tip teeth a small amount. The outer wire can also be adjusted for other small movements. Dr. Lanzetta says "small movements" because the best way to move a tooth is to firmly attach a brace to it, to create a secure handle. When a brace is glued right to a tooth, the doctor can intrude it, move it left, move it right, erupt it, rotate, spin it, and angle it. Dr. Lanzetta does not have nearly this much control with a finger spring. Since the movements available with a Hawley involve simply tipping teeth, the range of movements is very limited.

Recently Dr. Lanzetta has been adding fun designs and graphics to Hawley retainers. He starts by printing out logos, icons, sports team mascots and characters, then he adds them to the retainer. Kids love this. They can also add one or more custom colors to the acrylic. Do you love the Detroit Tigers? Then Dr. Lanzetta can make your retainer orange and blue. Want a rainbow? How about sparkles – they have gold and silver. Allowing patients to choose the style of their retainers has really added fun to the process of retention.

The disadvantages of this retainer are size and wear time. Since this retainer is somewhat thicker, people are often unhappy with how it immediately feels. Your speech will be impacted, and it will just feel thick. As one of Dr. Lanzetta's dental school instructors used to say, "It feels like you have the whole courthouse steps in your mouth." But like anything else, with time you will adjust to it. In fact, with proper and consistent wear, it's remarkable how unnoticeable it becomes.

The trick to success with a Hawley is to fully commit to it by wearing it full-time.

Because it does not contact each tooth as intimately as other retainers, it has to be worn for more hours per day. Typically Dr. Lanzetta recommends 20 to 22 hours of wear for the first year. This can be challenging for families, and it takes a focused commitment. Like brushing your teeth or wearing contacts, proper wear of your retainers becomes a part of your routine and daily life. Dr. Lanzetta believes that the best way to approach the wearing of a Hawley is to simply wear it full-out, as close to 22 hours a day as possible. Do not take it out when in public or when on the phone. This will force you to learn how to adjust to it, and before you know it, it will feel essentially invisible.

Essix

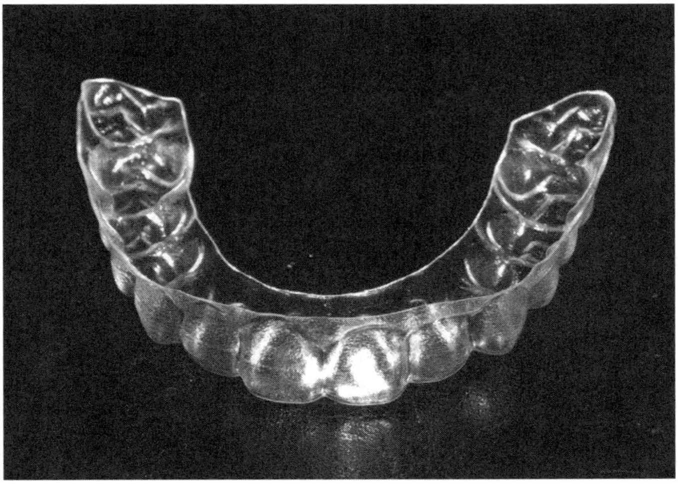

Essix retainers are thin, clear plastic retainers that are vacu-formed to a model of your teeth to form a perfect custom second skin covering your teeth. Essix retainers have a different set of advantages, including comfort, fit and control, protection of teeth, and wear time.

The advantages of an Essix retainer are its comfort and wear time. They are so thin that after just a few days of wearing them, they almost feel like you are not even wearing a retainer. Most people adapt to these retainers very quickly. Because they form such a close and custom fit to your teeth, they are only needed 12 hours per day. This is a huge advantage since with this wear pattern, they do not need to be removed from the home. This means less chance of them being left behind at school or at a restaurant. No more dumpster diving! Don't get too complacent, though: around every corner is an eager garbage disposal, toilet or puppy dog just dying to consume your beautiful Essix. You still have to exercise good judgment in taking care of your Essix.

They are not as durable as Hawleys, and in fact, will simply wear out at some point. If broken, they cannot be repaired. Essix retainers will typically last about one to two years and that is it. How much you grind your teeth at night, how acidic your saliva is, and how you brush them will be determining factors as to how long they will last. Dr. Lanzetta has had the occasional four-year-old Essix survive, but that is quite rare – it is like getting 70,000 miles on a set of 50,000-mile tires.

If you tend to clench or grind your teeth in your sleep, you will wear out an Essix much quicker. Small holes will start to develop, then small tears and cracks, until eventually it is no longer serviceable. Since this behavior occurs during sleep, it is not something that most people can voluntarily cease. Because of this, for those who quickly and aggressively wear down this retainer, they will probably have to switch to a Hawley at some point. Some patients choose the strategy to start off with an Essix until it wears out, then switch over to a Hawley. This way, they sort of get the best of both worlds: The advantage of night-time-only wear to start, followed by the advantage of a durable retainer later.

Essix are less adjustable. Because of their physical composition, there is little that Dr. Lanzetta can do to modify them. He can place small bumps or divots in the acrylic using specialized pliers. The divots place a small amount of pressure on strategic spots on teeth for minor movements. He can also make small adjustments to the teeth when it's first manufactured. He does this by adjusting the position or shape of the teeth on the model before the Essix is vacu-formed. Traditionally this was done on a plaster model by shaving off the plaster on one side of a tooth and adding wax to the other side of the tooth. The "scratch-and-fill" method gives the orthodontist a chance to add pressure to a particular part of a tooth. Another way to do this is to actually cut off the tooth from the plaster model, then literally move the plaster tooth into the desired position, and then make the Essix.

This entire process is now done digitally, and is the high-tech way that Invisalign® is made. A digital scan of your teeth is assembled in a computer, then the computer image of the tooth is moved in much the same way the actual plaster tooth is moved. The digital model is then printed at an outside lab with a 3-D printer, and an Essix made from this model. In the very near future, most orthodontic offices will have the equipment in their offices to be able to digitally scan your teeth and then use their own 3-D printer to make a model of your teeth and then make retainers. The future is very exiting.

Bonded Lingual

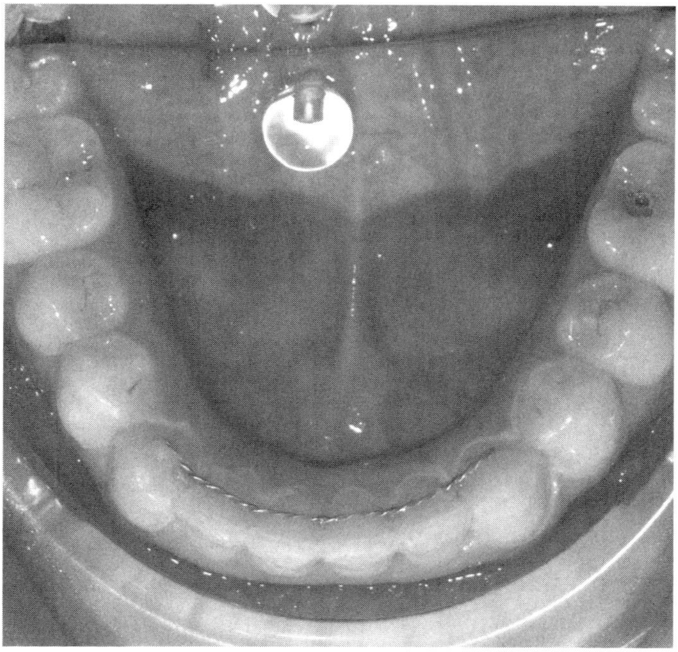

A bonded-lingual retainer is a wire that is bonded or glued on to the lingual surface of the teeth. Dr. Lanzetta usually bonds this wire to the front six lower teeth. The teeth are prepared much like they would be for getting braces glued on, except the wire is glued directly to the lingual surface of the lower front teeth. A small blob of clear acrylic glue is placed right over the wire and onto the tooth – no braces are used, just the wire and the acrylic glue. The wire and the acrylic work together to hold teeth in place.

For reasons that will be very clear, this retainer is a frequently requested item in our office. Imagine that you never have to nag your child to put his/her retainer in! This retainer is the dream of moms and dads the world over. Within a week or two, you can't even tell it's in your mouth. It is very comfortable, and does its magic all by itself.

So what's not to love? Two things: One, it becomes almost impossible to floss. The wire blocks your attempts to get the floss all the way down the contact point between the two teeth. Dental hygienists are not super huge fans of this retainer. Two, it can break loose. If it breaks loose, teeth can move. When this unfortunate event happens, too often the patient doesn't notice it, and the teeth experience considerable relapse. At this point, a patient's only recourse is additional treatment, obviously a frustrating and expensive situation. Further, it is possible that the acrylic glue becomes loose and you don't know it. If this happens, there is a very real fear that you will get decay underneath the glue as it is impossible to clean beneath it. This decay potential is significant, as most people have no idea that the glue came loose, and the decay can continue to cause extensive damage to the tooth. For most people, after a year or two of wearing a bonded-lingual retainer, they become unaware that they even have it.

A version of this bonded-lingual retainer is sometimes used on the front two upper teeth. Here's why: have you ever seen someone with a gap between their two front teeth? Think about Madonna, Elton John or Dave Letterman. These gaps are common. Closing that gap is easy with braces, but keeping it closed is challenging. The space is VERY tenacious. As soon as you take your retainer out, the space tries to creep back open. By bonding a wire, orthodontists can overcome this persistent problem. The same advantages and disadvantages exist with this smaller limited version.

WHEN DO I HAVE TO WEAR RETAINERS AND FOR HOW LONG?

It is often said in dentistry, "Only brush the teeth you want to keep." Well, in the world of retention, orthodontists say, "Only wear a retainer when you want your teeth to stay straight." There is simply no way around it. And the simplest way to put it is, if you wear retainers after braces or Invisalign®, your teeth will stay straight, and if you don't, they won't. It really is almost just that simple. But you may ask why or for how long? Must patients wear a retainer all day for the rest of their lives? Technically, yes, but this is not reasonable or practical. Instead, let's devise a protocol that safely retains teeth in position with a minimum of effort and time.

There are two main categories of why teeth move or relapse. Orthodontic relapse and Maturational relapse. Orthodontic relapse occurs after moving teeth with braces and Maturational relapse occurs whether or not you had braces. Here is the explanation about how teeth move with braces, and that will help with an understanding of these two processes.

HOW TEETH MOVE WITH BRACES

Contrary to the way you might think about it, teeth are not cemented into the bone. Think about it. If teeth couldn't move, Dr. Lanzetta would probably be a dentist instead of an orthodontist.

Although teeth feel so very tight and permanent, the position of your teeth is very dynamic. They are held in position by millions of tiny connective tissue fibers called Periodontal Fibers that surround it. These fibers are similar to the connective tissue fibers that hold your skin to your bones. A tooth is held to the bone by the root. The surface of the root does not touch the bone. Instead, it is suspended. If you look carefully, when you push on a tooth, it moves. It gives a little. The movement is fibers stretching or compacting. When you push on a tooth in one direction, the fibers on the side you push get stretched, and the fibers on the opposite side get compressed. Orthodontists know this, and they can even see it under a microscope. Fibers that are compressed send a signal to the cells in the area to start dissolving bone so that the tooth can move in that direction. The fibers on the opposite side get stretched, and as a result, other cells are signaled to make more bone. In this way, the leading edge of the tooth dissolves bone while the opposite side makes new bone, and the tooth slowly moves along.

At all times, it is the fibers that allow the process to happen. In fact, there is a disease process called ankylosis which involves a breakdown of the fiber system. The roots of the teeth do not have fibers, and instead touch the bone directly. In ankylosis, teeth cannot and will not move, at all. It follows then that these fibers that are responsible for tooth movement are also responsible for the relapse. Once a tooth has been moved into its position, what remains are millions of fibers that are still stretched.

Orthodontists know that the fibers remain under some amount of tension for years. And this is where orthodontic relapse comes from. Imagine pushing a tooth to the left for example. The fibers get stretched under tension and try to pull the tooth back to the right. There have been some studies that show that cutting those fibers released some of the tension and lessened some of the relapse.

Dr. Lanzetta is resistant to this "fiberotomy" procedure for a number of reasons. It is incomplete since you can't cut all the way down the root, it is painful and invasive, and it does not stop all relapse. In any event, the mouth is left with fibers that are under tension – and orthodontists have to take measures to control it, namely, you guessed it. Retainers.

Orthodontic relapse is the relapse that occurs from remaining tension from periodontal fibers. It is most strongly seen right after orthodontic tooth movement and lessens with time. Orthodontists will use this fact to design a way of keeping teeth in place with the least amount of effort necessary.

Maturational relapse really isn't relapse. Dr. Lanzetta is using the term to compare it to Orthodontic relapse. Perhaps a better term would be Maturational changes or movements. As we age through our 30's and 40's and 50's and on, forces are at work. Various factors are influencing the positions of our teeth. Chewing forces, growth of the jaw bones, the lips and tongue, swallowing, and breathing all present pressures that act to change the mouth and teeth.

Back teeth have a slight forward tilt to them so that when we bite down, the crowns push forward toward the front teeth. Dr. Lanzetta suspects this is to keep the teeth tight together. This forward pressure is very light, but over the decades it can add up. The effect is to drive the back teeth forward into the front teeth and add pressure. Also, the upper teeth fit over the lower teeth like a lid on a cookie jar. The upper teeth then place yet another gentle but constant pressure on the lower teeth. Finally, the jaws themselves continue to very slowly grow and change even in our middle decades.

All of these normal maturational changes add up to place pressure on the front teeth. The pressure is manifested in an increase in crowding of the front teeth over time. It is well documented that, even in someone who never had braces, their front teeth will become more crowded and crooked with time.

So to summarize then, we have Orthodontic relapse and Maturational relapse. How do we tell them apart and how do we control them? The short answer is that we can't always fully tell them apart, but we can take reasonable steps to control them.

We now return to our original question: "When do I have to wear retainers and for how long?" Let's break this up into its two parts: how many hours per day, and for how many years.

HOURS PER DAY

Dr. Lanzetta recommends a different routine depending upon the original problem and which retainer is selected.

Shortly after braces are removed or your orthodontist is finished with Invisalign, the tension on the periodontal fibers is highest, and orthodontic relapse is strongest. This tension fades best *if* the teeth are held in position. That means that the more consistent you are with your retainers, the better they will be at holding your teeth in place. Restated, the better we hold teeth in place, the better and faster they become stable.

Obviously if a bonded retainer is used, it is worn completely full-time since it is glued right in. As we have talked about, the main advantage of this retainer is indeed the fact that you don't have to do anything. It just sits there beautifully and dutifully preventing teeth from moving.

For a Hawley, Dr. Lanzetta recommends full-time, 24 x 7 for the first year, then bedtime only as-needed. Dr. Lanzetta will explain the "as-needed" bit later on. When Dr. Lanzetta recommends a Hawley, the very best way to wear this retainer is simply all the time. It is a bit bigger and harder to adjust to, and so the best approach is to wear it as close to 24 hours a day as possible.

There are two times that you can and should remove them: eating and brushing. Other than that, Dr. Lanzetta has found that when people really full-out commit to wear them, they become easy. Just like new shoes or earrings or nearly anything else we do, the more we use something, the more normal it feels and the more invisible it becomes. This is a really important point and one Dr. Lanzetta often spends quite a bit of time on with patients. As soon as patients start having trouble with Hawley retainers, the first thing they want to do is to take them out and give themselves a break. That is the *last* thing you should do! If you can discipline yourself to gut it out, you will find that before you know it, you won't even notice that you have retainers in. At that point, usually within two weeks,

Hawley retainers become very simple and easy. Although it does take some work to get to this point it is well worth it.

In fact, this step is so important, you can often predict who will ultimately be successful with retainers. If you start off with the bad habit of taking out your retainers when you have to talk on the phone or when at work or school, you will always see your retainers as an obstacle and annoyance, and at some point you will likely give up. Remember, your teeth will not stay straight without retainers!

If you can manage to wear your Hawleys well for one year, you have earned the benefit of wearing them during bedtime hours only. At this point, the teeth are becoming more stable. The teeth will not move significantly during the 14 to 18 hours that they be without retainers. You will likely notice that at night when you go to place your retainers in, they are a little bit tight. This is normal. A small amount of movement is to be expected; and quite frankly, we will rarely be in the position where the teeth become so stable that they show no movement at all after a day of freedom. Let's be reasonable about this. If after a full day of leaving your retainers out, they feel just the tiniest bit tight, and the tightness only lasts for a minute, then we can safely assume that for the most part, your teeth are nicely stable.

Remember our goal: to devise a protocol that safely retains teeth in position with a minimum of effort and time. After a year of faithful full-time wear, most people are perfectly safe with wearing their Hawley retainers at bedtime, seven nights a week. Continue this practice for at least two to three more years.

For an Essix, Dr. Lanzetta recommends that they be worn immediately after dinner, until breakfast. In other words, from the time you finish dinner, say 7:00 p.m., all through the evening, then all through the night until morning. This usually amounts to about 10 to 12 hours. The following day, when you first put them back in, they will feel a little snug. This is normal, and will only last a few minutes as they settle back in.

The big question becomes, why do you only require 12 hours with an Essix when you require 24 hours with a Hawley? The reason comes down to fit. The way an Essix is designed, the plastic parts completely and intimately surrounds every single part of each tooth. The contact is better, more accurate, and more complete, and thus the retention is better. From all of my years of doing this, I have realized that for better or worse, a Hawley needs that full-time wear, whereas an Essix does not.

In a similar manner to Hawleys, after one year of faithful wear of Essix retainers, you can as well transition to wearing them during bedtime hours only. Again, you will likely find that they are mildly snug for a moment or two at bedtime when you first put them in.

OKAY, NOW HOW LONG DO I HAVE TO WEAR MY RETAINERS?

You may have heard it said that you have to wear retainers for the rest of your life, or that you have to wear retainers as long as you want your teeth to be straight. Technically, that's true. No orthodontist would ever argue that the most reliable way to prevent teeth from ever moving is to lock them down for life. However, in the real world, Dr.

Lanzetta does not think that that is very reasonable or realistic, and he feels that that is an insufficient way of dealing with the problem. He believes that if you tell a person that they will have to wear retainers for the rest of his/her lives, then you have removed any chance of helping to modify his/her behavior in a realistic and reasonable manner.

Here's how he recommends his patients manage this dilemma: wear your retainers so that they are not tight. That's it! Just don't let your retainers get tight.

What does this mean? Let's first think in terms of extremes. If you were to leave your retainers out for five seconds, when you put them back in, they will not be tight, right? The teeth have not had a chance to move. If you were to leave them out for five days, and your teeth did in fact move during those five days, when you put your retainers back in, they would feel tight. It's more likely that they would feel very tight! Think of the tightness as a signal that your teeth are sending you. They are yelling at you, "Hey, you, we have moved, and now that those retainers are back on us, we feel it!" When you think about it this way, there is a very simple system for knowing how long you have to wear your retainers for: wear them enough so that they are not tight when you put them back in.

In actuality, this will mean something different for every person. We are all completely unique individuals. No two person's teeth will stabilize at the same rate. Rather than use an arbitrary time period or schedule, Dr. Lanzetta simply tells patients to wear their retainers enough so that they are not tight. For some, they will be able to wear retainers for less than five years while for others they may have to wear them for more than 20 years.

Dr. Lanzetta can best summarize this by saying that by and large, for most people in most situations, it is safe to say that if properly worn, you will need to wear retainers for about five to 10 years, but your mileage may vary. I think this is a fair and acceptable proposition. Dr. Lanzetta worries that patients will give up prematurely due to a feeling of despair trying to reach a goal that is impossible to reach, rather he wants people to feel like they can see the finish line – and that our goal is attainable. Five to 10 years initially sounds like a long time, and it is, but it ends up going by fast, and it is certainly less time than "the rest of your life"!

For bonded-lingual retainers, Dr. Lanzetta recommends that they be removed after five years. This should be enough time to develop reasonably good stability. There is a concern that there could be damage or decay under the appliance if left any longer. Typically, after this retainer is removed, a Hawley or Essix is fabricated to ensure long-term stability. Even after wearing a bonded retainer for every second of every day for five years, yes, the teeth can still relapse. This is another reason Dr. Lanzetta doesn't routinely recommend this retainer: despite wearing it successfully for years, you still may need yet another retainer.

HOW RETAINERS ARE MADE

Hawley retainers are made of acrylic and metal wires. The wires are stainless steel, and the acrylic is a plastic made from a liquid and powder. When the liquid and powder parts of the resin plastic are mixed, it turns into a solid, clear plastic.

First, a model of the teeth is made. For decades this model was made out of plaster taken from an impression using dental alginate. As Dr. Lanzetta has mentioned, we now have the ability to make models out of plastic using a 3-D printer. A digital impression is made that creates a computer 3-D model of the teeth, like a CAD/CAM system. The virtual digital model is then printed out into a real plastic model with a 3-D printer. The wires are then bent and placed onto the teeth. This usually includes two wires: a wire that goes in front of the front six teeth, and a small wire that goes in the back (a clasp) that is used to hold the retainer in the mouth.

These wires are bent into position, and held onto the model using wax. The wire is held in place as melted wax is dripped onto the wire and onto the model. Once the wires are in place and steady, a small paintbrush is dipped into the liquid part of the acrylic, then dabbed into the powder. A thick but "flow-able" resin is created, about the consistency of warm molasses. This resin is "painted" onto the model bit by bit until the plastic part of the retainer is created. After about 10 minutes, the acrylic is fully cured, and the entire piece can be removed from the model, trimmed and polished. The finished product should be clear and smooth and without sharp edges.

Essix retainers are thin clear plastic shells that fit completely around all visible sides of the teeth, almost like a second skin. They also require a model of the teeth. The model is placed in a special device, called a vacu-form machine. This machine heats up a thin piece of plastic until it is quite soft. At the right moment, the plastic is quickly placed right over the model as a vacuum pulls the warm and flexible plastic over the teeth. The plastic conforms to the teeth and quickly hardens as it cools. It is then trimmed and polished.

There are two ways to make a lingual-bonded retainer: direct and indirect. The direct way is to pre-bend a small wire on the model of the teeth so that the wire follows along the inside surface of the front six lower teeth. The teeth are prepared in the same way they are prepared for braces, namely, they are cleaned and prepped using chemicals and adhesives. The wire is held in place as a small amount of acrylic adhesive is added over the wire. This acrylic is typically light-activated to harden it.

The indirect method is similar (only after the wire is pre-bent as in the direct way), and it is held in place on the model with a small amount of wax. Then a type of putty (about the consistency of Silly Putty) is placed over the wire and around the front six teeth. The putty is then removed after it hardens, with the wire held inside of it. The teeth are then prepared as before, and this time, the glue is added on the teeth first, then the wire and putty are placed onto the teeth. Indirect bonding can provide for better and more accurate placement of the wire, however there are many opportunities to make mistakes and if the entire process is not done just right, the wire retainer will not adapt properly and thus it will not do its job.

HOW TO DETERMINE WHICH TYPE OF RETAINER TO USE

There are two criteria for determining which of these three retainers would be the best one to use: features and performance.

Features

For the most part, the decision for which retainer to use will fall to the patient and family. After all, they are the ones who have to wear them, take care of them, and possibly replace them. Given the long list of different advantages, Dr. Lanzetta would prefer to explain the differences, and then let the family decide. As long as they understand the consequences of the different strengths and weaknesses of the different types, Dr. Lanzetta is content with them making the decision. In most cases, either of these types will work just fine and hold the teeth in position.

Performance

Dr. Lanzetta will often let patients choose which retainer they want to use. Given that the experience of wearing the different types of retainers and the disadvantages and costs can vary, Dr. Lanzetta prefers to let families decide what makes the most sense.

However, there are times when Dr. Lanzetta will encourage patients to use a particular one due to a special mechanical need or other advantage. For example, in some cases, it is important that the teeth do not touch each other during sleep. Some people clench their jaws and teeth together, which causes wear, muscle soreness, and headaches. This situation calls for an Essix retainer as the plastic covers over the biting surfaces of the teeth and does not allow them to touch or wear.

Also, one particular type of problem, an open bite, is better retained with an Essix. Due to the fact that the Essix is better at grabbing the entire surface of the incisors, it can better resist them from relapsing back into an open bite. A Hawley may be the retainer of choice for someone who squeezes tightly on their teeth and quickly wears out or cracks and destroys an Essix retainer. That patient is better off going with a Hawley (which will last much longer) or an appliance called a Bite Splint, which is a much thicker and stronger acrylic plate that your dentist makes. It is not economical to have to replace an Essix every six months because you are chewing through it.

CARING FOR RETAINERS

As Dr. Lanzetta has mentioned, proper care and use of retainers should prove years of use. You will notice that since they are in your mouth for a considerable amount of time, if left alone, they will quickly become dirty, smelly, and covered in plaque and calculus (tartar, a hard substance formed when calcium from the saliva hardens plaque). The best way to correct this problem is to prevent it from happening in the first place.

Dr. Lanzetta recommends patients brush their retainers as if their retainer was another tooth. That's right, simple toothbrush and toothpaste. Start a daily routine of always brushing your retainers whenever you brush your teeth and they will never have a chance to accumulate plaque and calculus. They will last longer, look better and smell better.

Contrary to popular myth, you do not have to soak retainers in water. If you leave them out of your mouth, simply keep them in your case. If they are picking up an odor, it is reasonable to soak them in a mint mouth rinse such as

Listerine. We have found that there is no advantage to soaking retainers in an effervescent powder such as Polident – the retainers end up no cleaner than if you would have simply brushed them with toothpaste.

A word of caution: *retainers are plastic*. They will melt under extreme heat of a toaster or an oven, but more importantly, they will distort under the moderate heat of a clothes dryer, dishwasher or car dashboard in the summer. Be careful not to expose your retainers to very warm or hot temperatures.

Retainers are the favorite toys of dogs. For some strange reason, dogs just love these things. They smell them out and find them. Dr. Lanzetta has had countless retainers brought back to the office after Fido or Rex had gotten hold of it. And once the dog gets it, the retainer is all but unrecognizable. Even the top of your dresser or kitchen counter is not safe. Dogs will find a way to get them. Keep them safe and in your case and far away from your dog.

If a retainer breaks, please come into the office within two weeks. DR. LANZETTA CANNOT EMPHASIZE THIS ENOUGH. If a retainer is lost or broken, do yourself a favor and call us right away. Do not wait. Sadly, almost every month a patient returns to our office three to six months after being unable to wear a retainer. Typically, the teeth have moved so much that they need some form of treatment again. This is very frustrating and very expensive. No one wants to go through treatment again and certainly no one want to pay for it again, but we do lead very busy lives. Dr. Lanzetta understands that. But please take these words seriously and remember to call and return to your orthodontist's office right away. You will be glad you did.

When you first are fitted with your retainers, Dr. Lanzetta will ask that you return in about four weeks for a check. He will evaluate how the retainer fits, how it performs, if any teeth have moved, and overall how you are doing with it. If all goes well, Dr. Lanzetta will schedule a six-month retainer check. At this point, things are going well, and you have established a routine.

As previously noted, if you notice a tooth moving, if you have cracked or damaged or broken a retainer, or if you are just uncertain about something, do not wait. Call and come in within two weeks. Dr. Lanzetta will check to make sure everything is okay and take the necessary steps to ensure that your teeth are being held properly. He will then continue to see you for another two years or so. By this time, you are very aware of how well your retainers fit. At all times, you are the doctor's patient.. That means you are always welcome to return for any reason or any question. Some of his patients return once a year, like the Swallows of Capistrano, just to say hi and renew the friendship that was started way back when treatment first started. He and his staff love seeing their old friends. You are always welcome.

CONCLUSION

It is difficult to describe the wonderful feelings people get the day they are done straightening their teeth. There is just nothing quite like a beautiful smile and the joy and satisfaction of having a wonderful smile after going through orthodontic treatment. Keeping your teeth straight for as long as you want them straight is absolutely possible and is completely up to you. We are here to straighten your teeth, and we are here to help you keep them straight.

It may seem like a tedious, long and frustrating burden to have to wear retainers for such a long time, but in reality, when done properly and as Dr. Lanzetta recommends, the retention experience can be easy and simple. Dr. Lanzetta wants you to love your smile, and he wants you to keep your smile for a lifetime. Dr. Lanzetta is fortunate to be able to provide people with a great, healthy smile, and it is very satisfying and rewarding to have a career such as this. But Dr. Lanzetta gets just as much satisfaction when he sees a patient eight or 10 years later with wonderful straight teeth, who has overcome relapse with a simple, properly worn retainer.